The DASH Diet

Over 100 recipes for breakfast, lu

By Susan Evans

Copyright © 2015 Susan Evans

All rights reserved. This book or any portion thereof may not be reproduced or used in any manner whatsoever without the express written permission of the publisher except for the use of brief quotations in a book review.

Other popular books by Susan Evans

Vegetarian Mediterranean Cookbook:
Over 50 recipes for appetizers, salads, dips, and main dishes

Quick & Easy Asian Vegetarian Cookbook:
Over 50 recipes for stir fries, rice, noodles, and appetizers

Vegetarian Slow Cooker Cookbook:
Over 75 recipes for meals, soups, stews, desserts, and sides

Quick & Easy Vegan Desserts Cookbook:
Over 80 delicious recipes for cakes, cupcakes, brownies, cookies, fudge, pies, candy, and so much more!

Quick & Easy Microwave Meals:
Over 50 recipes for breakfast, snacks, meals and desserts

Quick & Easy Vegetarian Rice Cooker Meals:
Over 50 recipes for breakfast, main dishes, and desserts

Quick & Easy Rice Cooker Meals:
Over 60 recipes for breakfast, main dishes, soups, and desserts

Halloween Cookbook:
80 Ghoulish recipes for appetizers, meals, drinks, and desserts

Free Bonus!

Would you like to receive one of my cookbooks for free? Just leave me on honest review on Amazon and I will send you a digital version of the cookbook of your choice! All you have to do is email me proof of your review and the desired cookbook and format to susan.evans.author@gmail.com. Thank you for your support, and have fun cooking!

Introduction 1

Measurement Conversions 3

Breakfast 4

Chicken Parmesan and Baked Quinoa 5
Raisins, Apples, and Cinnamon Granola 7
Mushroom Strata and Turkey Sausage Casserole.........8
Blueberry-Raspberry Mint Gazpacho............................9
Very Berry Muesli 10
Avocado, Banana & Chocolate Pudding......................11
Banana-Oatmeal Pancake with Spiced Maple Syrup ..12
Breakfast Bread Pudding..14
Veggie Quiche Muffins 15
Cheese Broccoli Mini Egg Omelettes 16
Peanut Butter & Banana Breakfast Smoothie..............17
Baked Apple Spice Oatmeal 18
Strawberry Tapioca 19
Strawberry Salad with Balsamic Vinegar......................20
Blueberry Steel Cut Oat Pancakes with Agave 21

Lunch 22

Buffalo Chicken Salad Wrap 23
Chicken sliders 24
Tuna Melt 25
*Curried Garbanzo Beans and Mustard Greens with
Sweet Potatoes* 26
*Roasted Brussel Sprouts and Caramelized Butternut
Squash with Quinoa*..27

Turkey, Pear, and Cheese Sandwich 28
Salmon Salad Pita 29
Turkey Apple Gyro 30
Southwest Style Rice Bowl 31
Sunshine Wrap 32
Tuna Pita Pockets 33

SALADS 34

Citrus Salad 35
Raw Kale Salad with Lemon Tahini Dressing 36
Black Bean Southwest Salad 38
Mediterranean Tuna Salad 39
Tangy Mango Salad 40
Winter Citrus Salad 41
Pineapple Chicken Salad with Balsamic Vinaigrette .. 42
Grilled Chicken Avocado and Mango Salad 43
Southwestern Black Bean Cakes with Guacamole 44
Almond Chicken Pear Salad 45
Curried Garbanzo Beans and Mustard Greens with Sweet Potatoes 46
Mango Curry Chicken Salad 47
Avocado Salad with Ginger-Miso Dressing 48
Spring Nicoise Potato Salad 49
Strawberries, Blue Cheese, and Chicken Mixed Greens Salad with Poppy Seed Dressing 50
Shrimp, Strawberry and Feta Salad 51
Apricot Chicken Pasta Salad 52
Crispy Citrus Salad with Grilled Cod 53
Cinnamon Pistachio Chicken Salad 54
Rocket and Veggie Ham Salad 55

SOUPS 56

Ginger Chicken Noodle Soup 57
Autumn Squash Ginger Bisque 58
Potato Soup with Brie Cheese and Apple 59
Greek Lentil Soup 60
Leftover Turkey Chili 61
Roasted Pear and Squash Soup 62
Curried Carrot Soup 63
Wild Rice Mushroom Soup 64
Seafood Chowder 65
Spicy Chili Soup 66
Shamrock Soup 67
Steamy Salmon Chowder 68

DINNER 69

Grilled Pineapple Salsa Beef Kabobs 70
Sesame-Honey Chicken and Quinoa 72
Shrimp Pasta Primavera 73
Chicken Pesto Bake 74
Grilled Chicken with Crunchy Apple Salsa 75
Curried Pork in Apple Cider 76
Halibut with Tomato and Basil Salsa 77
Cranberry Chicken 78
Whiskey-Mushroom New York Strip Steak 79
Pear Curry Chicken 80
Mustard-Dill Poached Salmon 81
Fish Cod Fillet Tacos 82
Garlic and Lime Pork Chops 83
Honey Crusted Chicken 84
Spicy Mango Jerk Chicken 85

Lemon Chicken and Potatoes 86
Pork Medallions with Herbes de Provence 87
Pork Tenderloin with Apples and Balsamic Vinegar...88
Salsa Verde Burger 89
Brazilian Black Beans Sausage 90
Tangy Yogurt Broiled Halibut 91
Mediterranean-Style Grilled Salmon................................92
Chicken with Oranges and Avocados 93
Lime and Cilantro Tilapia Tacos......................................94
Sesame Baked Chicken Tenders..95
Spicy Pork with Sweet Potatoes and Apples 96
Glazed Turkey Breast with Fruit Stuffing......................98
Pork Chops with Black Currant Sauce 100
Honey Mustard Grilled Chicken with Toasted Almonds 101
Grilled Pesto Shrimp Skewers...102
Grilled Pork Fajitas...103
Southeast Asian Baked Salmon......................................104
Grilled Snapper Curry..105
Roasted Salmon with Maple Glaze 106
Spinach, Shrimp and Feta with Tuscan White Beans 107

DESSERTS 108

Red, White, and Blue Fruit Skewers and Cheesecake Dip..109
Honey and Yogurt Grilled Peaches 110
Blackberry Cinnamon Ginger Iced Tea 111
Apples and Cream Shake 112
Fruited Rice Pudding 113

SNACKS AND SIDES..........................114

Sweet and Spicy Roasted Red Pepper Hummus.........115
Chipotle Spiced Shrimp..................................116
Lemon Glaze..117
Maple Mustard Kale with Turkey Bacon 118
Garlic and Kale with Black-Eyed Peas.......................119
Sweet and Spicy Snack Mix 120
Baked Pears with Walnuts and Honey.......................121
Classic Boston Baked Beans................................122
Grilled Mango Chutney....................................123
Sherried Mushroom Sauce 124
Bulgur Stuffing with Dried Cranberries and Hazelnuts125
Southwest Potato Skins 127
Shrimp ceviche 128

THANK YOU 129

INTRODUCTION

You are about to revolutionize your eating habits and it is going to be a life changing experience! If you have been suffering from hypertension (high blood pressure) or just want to start eating healthier and don't quite know what meals you need to introduce to your diet, worry no more. It's time to put the DASH in your diet and celebrate a healthy eating regime that it is highly recommended by medical and nutritional professionals and has been named the #1 leading diet by US News & World since 2011 for four consecutive years! DASH stands for **D**ietary **A**pproaches to **S**top **H**ypertension and has been intensively researched, coupled by scientific studies that show that it is the best diet towards hypertension and for anyone wanting to live a healthy lifestyle.

You have probably had the displeasure of experiencing conventional diet plans that restrict you from eating delicious and scrumptious meals. Why should you have to live through boring and flavorless food? Here is the fun part - this DASH Diet cookbook does not subscribe to that bland plan! Getting the right nutrition as well as visually admiring your artistic food is going to be the order of the day when it comes to the DASH Diet.

I have put together this handy and useful cookbook full of recipes compiled according to the endorsements of the DASH Diet. It contains many delicious recipes and mouth-watering meal plans that will make cooking fun and easy; whilst helping you to maintain good health. Foods such as processed can-foods, junk food, high fat items are highly discouraged. Whereas, home-cooked meals with fresh vegetables and fresh meat, and non-processed foods are highly welcomed and most certainly celebrated. This Dash Diet cookbook unlocks many recipes that encourage healing to take place in your body. Following these delectable, lip-smacking well thought-out healthy recipes will encourage an enjoyable lifestyle.

This cookbook contains a complete diet plan which includes tasty morning breakfast delights, healthy lunch meals, tasty snacks, savory soups, delicious salads, delectable dinner recipes, and of course desserts! Instructions and guidelines are simple and allow for a very easy, step by step meal preparation plan. Prepare yourself for a magical taste-bud adventure whilst your body starts regenerating itself and facilitating wellbeing at the same time. You know the drill, let's drop the bad eating habits, add a DASH of wonderment and let's get cooking!

MEASUREMENT CONVERSIONS

Liquid/Volume Measurements (approximate)

1 teaspoon = 1/6 fluid ounce (oz.) = 1/3 tablespoon = 5 ml

1 tablespoon = 1/2 fluid ounce (oz.) = 3 teaspoons = 15 ml

1 fluid ounce (oz.) = 2 tablespoons = 1/8 cup = 30 ml

1/4 cup = 2 fluid ounces (oz.) = 4 tablespoons = 60 ml

1/3 cup = 2⅔ fluid ounces (oz.) = 5 ⅓ tablespoons = 80 ml

1/2 cup = 4 fluid ounces (oz.) = 8 tablespoons = 120 ml

2/3 cup = 5⅓ fluid ounces (oz.) = 10⅔ tablespoons = 160 ml

3/4 cup = 6 fluid ounces (oz.) = 12 tablespoons = 180 ml

7/8 cup = 7 fluid ounces (oz.) = 14 tablespoons = 210 ml

1 cup = 8 fluid ounces (oz.) = 1/2 pint = 240 ml

1 pint = 16 fluid ounces (oz.) = 2 cups = 1/2 quart = 475 ml

1 quart = 4 cups = 32 fluid ounces (oz.) = 2 pints = 950 ml

1 liter = 1.055 quarts = 4.22 cups = 2.11 pints = 1000 ml

1 gallon = 4 quarts = 8 pints = 3.8 liters

Dry/Weight Measurements (approximate)

1 ounce (oz.) = 30 grams (g)

2 ounces (oz.) = 55 grams (g)

3 ounces (oz.) = 85 grams (g)

1/4 pound (lb.) = 4 ounces (oz.) = 125 grams (g)

1/2 pound (lb.) = 8 ounces (oz.) = 240 grams (g)

3/4 pound (lb.) = 12 ounces (oz.) = 375 grams (g)

1 pound (lb.) = 16 ounces (oz.) = 455 grams (g)

2 pounds (lbs.) = 32 ounces (oz.) = 910 grams (g)

1 kilogram (kg) = 2.2 pounds (lbs.) = 1000 gram (g)

BREAKFAST

Chicken Parmesan and Baked Quinoa

SERVINGS: 6
PREP TIME: 20 min.
TOTAL TIME: 1 hour

Ingredients

- 1 tablespoon olive oil
- 1 medium onion, diced
- 3 cloves garlic, minced
- 2 tablespoon balsamic vinegar
- 1 (15 oz.) can tomato sauce
- 1 (15 oz.) can diced tomatoes (no added salt)
- basil and oregano, to taste
- 1 cup quinoa
- 2 cups water or broth
- 1 lb. boneless, skinless chicken, cooked and cut into bite sized pieces
- 2/3 cup shredded part-skim mozzarella cheese, divided
- 2 tablespoon grated Parmesan or Romano cheese

Instructions

1. Preheat the oven to 375°F (190°C) and spray a 2 quart baking dish with cooking oil.
2. Heat a large skillet over medium heat and add oil. Stir in onion. Stir frequently for about 5-7 minutes, or until tender. Add garlic and cook until fragrant, about 30-60 seconds. Add the balsamic vinegar, mix and cook until it is nearly fully absorbed.
3. Add tomato sauce, diced tomatoes, basil, oregano, and pepper to taste. Bring to a low boil and then simmer while you make the rest of the meal.
4. Place quinoa in a mesh strainer. Rinse with cold water for 2 minutes.
5. In a small sauce pan, place quinoa and water or broth and bring to a boil (add a little salt if using water). Cover with a lid, reduce heat, and simmer until cooked, around 20-25 minutes.

6. Combine and mix the quinoa and chicken with the sauce in a large bowl.
7. Place mix in the baking dish and top with the mozzarella cheese and Parmesan.
8. Cover with foil and bake for about 15 minutes.
9. Remove foil and bake until cheese is bubbly and lightly browned, about 10 more minutes.

Raisins, Apples, and Cinnamon Granola

SERVINGS: 12
PREP TIME: 15 min.
TOTAL TIME: 1 hour

Ingredients

- 1/4 cup slivered almonds
- 1/4 cup honey
- 1/4 cup unsweetened applesauce
- 1 tablespoon vanilla extract
- 1 tablespoon ground cinnamon
- 2 cups dry old-fashioned oatmeal
- 2 cups bran flakes
- 3/4 cup dried apple pieces
- 1/2 cup golden raisins

Instructions

1. Preheat the oven to 325°F (165°C). Lightly coat baking sheet with cooking spray.
2. Spread almonds on a baking sheet and bake. Stir occasionally for about 10 minutes, or until golden and fragrant. Transfer to a plate and cool. Raise temperature of the oven to 350°F (175°C).
3. In a small bowl, whisk honey, applesauce, vanilla and cinnamon together. Set aside.
4. Add oatmeal and bran flakes in a large bowl. Stir and mix well. Add honey mix and toss, being careful not to break the clumps apart.
5. Spread cereal mix evenly onto a baking sheet. Place in oven and stir occasionally. Bake until golden brown, about 30 minutes. Remove from oven and slightly cool.
6. Combine cereal mix, toasted almonds, apple pieces and raisins in a large bowl. Cool completely and store in an airtight container.

Mushroom Strata and Turkey Sausage Casserole

SERVINGS: 12
PREP TIME: 15 min.
TOTAL TIME: 1 hour + refrigeration

Ingredients

- 8 ounces wheat ciabatta bread, cut into 1-inch cubes
- 12 ounces turkey sausage
- 2 cups fat free milk
- 1-1/2 cup (4 ounces) reduced-fat shredded sharp cheddar cheese
- 3 large eggs
- 12 ounces egg substitute
- 1/2 cup chopped green onion
- 1 cup sliced mushrooms
- 1/2 teaspoon paprika
- Fresh ground pepper, to taste
- 2 tablespoons grated parmesan cheese

Instructions

1. Preheat oven to 400°F (200°C).
2. Arrange bread cubes on a baking sheet. Bake at 400°F (200°C) until toasted for about 8 minutes.
3. Heat a medium skillet over medium-high heat. Add sausage and cook 7 minutes or until browned. Stir to crumble.
4. In a large bowl combine milk, cheese, eggs, egg substitute, parmesan cheese, paprika, salt and pepper. Stir with a whisk.
5. Add bread, sausage, scallions and mushrooms. Toss well to coat bread. Spoon mix into a 13x9-inch baking dish. Cover and refrigerate for overnight or 8 hours.
6. Preheat oven to 350°F (175°C).
7. Uncover the casserole and bake for 50 minutes or until lightly browned.
8. Cut into 12 pieces and serve.

Blueberry-Raspberry Mint Gazpacho

SERVINGS: 4
PREP TIME: 5 min.
TOTAL TIME: 15 min. + refrigeration

Ingredients

- 1 1/2 cups blueberries
- 1 1/2 cups raspberries
- 2 tablespoons sugar
- 1 tablespoon orange juice
- 1 teaspoon lemon juice
- 1 teaspoon lime juice
- 1 teaspoon lemon zest
- Fresh mint leaves, for garnish
- 4 scoops (1/4 cup each) fat-free Greek yogurt

Instructions

1. In a medium heatproof bowl, combine berries, sugar, orange, lemon and lime juice, and lemon zest.
2. Cover bowl with plastic wrap.
3. Place bowl over a large saucepan of simmering water and cook 10 minutes on low.
4. Set aside until it cools and refrigerate for about 4 hours.
5. Divide fruit and its liquid among 4 bowls. Garnish with fresh mint and top each with a 1/4 cup scoop of Greek yogurt.

Very Berry Muesli

SERVINGS: 4
PREP/TOTAL TIME: 10 min. + refrigeration

Ingredients

- 1 cup old-fashioned rolled oats (raw)
- 1 cup fruit yogurt
- 1/2 cup 1% milk
- Pinch of salt
- 1/2 cup dried fruit (raisins, apricots, dates)
- 1/2 cup chopped apple
- 1/2 cup frozen blueberries
- 1/4 cup chopped, toasted walnuts

Instructions

1. Mix oats, yogurt, milk and salt in medium bowl.
2. Cover and refrigerate overnight.
3. Add dried and fresh fruit. Mix gently.
4. Serve scoops of muesli in small dishes and sprinkle each serving with chopped nuts.
5. Refrigerate leftovers within 2-3 hours.

Avocado, Banana & Chocolate Pudding

SERVINGS: 6
PREP TIME: 10 min.
TOTAL TIME: 1 hour 10 min

Ingredients

- 1 ripe avocado, peeled and pitted
- 4 very ripe bananas
- 1/4 cup unsweetened cocoa powder, plus more for garnish

Instructions

1. In a blender, blend avocados, bananas, and cocoa powder until smooth.
2. Pour into serving bowls and sprinkle additional cocoa powder on top.
3. Chill in refrigerator for at least 1 hour. Serve.

Banana-Oatmeal Pancake with Spiced Maple Syrup

SERVINGS: 6
PREP TIME: 10 min.
TOTAL TIME: 20 min.

Ingredients

- 1/2 cup maple syrup
- 1/2 cinnamon stick
- 3 whole cloves
- 1/2 cup old-fashioned rolled oats
- 1 cup water
- 2 tablespoons firmly packed light brown sugar
- 2 tablespoons canola oil
- 1/2 cup whole-wheat/whole-meal flour
- 1/2 cup all-purpose plain flour
- 1 1/2 teaspoons baking powder
- 1/4 teaspoon baking soda
- 1/4 teaspoon salt
- 1/4 teaspoon ground cinnamon
- 1/2 cup 1 percent low-fat milk
- 1/4 cup fat-free plain yogurt
- 1 banana, peeled and mashed
- 1 egg, lightly beaten

Instructions

1. In a small saucepan, combine maple syrup, cinnamon stick and cloves. Place over medium heat and bring to a boil. Remove heat and let stand for 15 minutes. Remove the cinnamon stick and cloves with a slotted spoon and set syrup aside. Keep warm.
2. Combine oats and water in a large microwave-safe bowl. Microwave on high about 3 minutes or until oats are creamy and tender. Stir in the brown sugar and canola oil. Set aside to slightly cool.

3. Combine flours, baking powder, baking soda, salt and ground cinnamon in a bowl. Whisk to blend.
4. Add milk, yogurt and banana to oats and stir until well mixed. Beat in the egg. Add flour mix to the oat mix and stir just until moistened.
5. Heat a non-stick frying pan or griddle over medium heat. Spoon 1/4 cup pancake batter into the pan. Cook until the top of pancake is covered with bubbles and the edges are slightly browned, about 2 minutes. Turn and cook until the bottom is well browned and the pancake is cooked through, about 1 to 2 more minutes. Repeat with the remaining pancake batter.
6. Place pancakes on warmed individual plates. Drizzle with the warm syrup and serve.

Breakfast Bread Pudding

SERVINGS: 4
PREP TIME: 10 min.
TOTAL TIME: 1 hour

Ingredients

- 1 1/2 cup low fat or fat free milk
- 4 eggs
- 2 tablespoons brown sugar
- 1/2 teaspoon vanilla extract
- 1/2 teaspoon ground cinnamon
- 1/8 teaspoon salt
- 3 cups cubed whole wheat bread, about 4 slices
- 1/2 cup peeled and diced apple
- 1/4 cup raisins
- 2 teaspoons powdered sugar (optional)

Instructions

1. Preheat oven to 350°F (175°C).
2. Combine milk, eggs, brown sugar, vanilla, cinnamon and salt in a large bowl. Whisk until combined.
3. Add bread cubes, diced apple and raisins, and mix until all ingredients are combined and bread has soaked up most of the liquid.
4. Coat an 8-inch square baking dish with butter or non-stick spray.
5. Transfer bread mixture into the baking pan. Cover with foil.
6. Place bread pudding into the oven and bake for 40 minutes. Uncover and continue baking until golden brown, about 20 minutes more.
7. Let stand for 10 minutes before serving. Dust with powdered sugar, if desired.

Veggie Quiche Muffins

SERVINGS: 12
PREP TIME: 10 min.
TOTAL TIME: 45 min.

Ingredients

- 3/4 cup low-fat cheddar cheese, shredded
- 1 cup green onion or onion, chopped
- 1 cup broccoli, chopped
- 1 cup tomatoes, diced
- 2 cups non-fat or 1% milk
- 4 eggs
- 1 cup baking mix (for biscuits or pancakes)
- 1 teaspoon Italian seasoning (or dried leaf basil and oregano)
- 1/2 teaspoon salt
- 1/2 teaspoon pepper

Instructions

1. Heat oven to 375°F (190°C) and lightly spray or oil 12 muffin cups.
2. Sprinkle cheese, onions, broccoli and tomatoes in muffin cups.
3. In a bowl, place remaining ingredients and beat until smooth. Pour egg mix over other ingredients in muffin cups.
4. Bake until golden brown, about 35-40 minutes or until knife inserted in center comes out clean. Cool 5 minutes.
5. Refrigerate leftovers.

Cheese Broccoli Mini Egg Omelettes

SERVINGS: 9
PREP TIME: 10 min.
TOTAL TIME: 40 min.

Ingredients

- 4 cups broccoli florets
- 4 whole eggs
- 1 cup egg whites
- 1/4 cup reduced fat cheddar
- 1/4 cup grated Romano or parmesan cheese
- 1 tablespoon olive oil
- salt and fresh pepper
- cooking spray

Instructions

1. Preheat oven to 350°F (175°C). Steam broccoli with some water for 6-7 minutes.
2. When broccoli is cooked, mash into smaller pieces. Add olive oil, salt and pepper. Mix well.
3. Spray muffin tin with cooking spray and spoon broccoli mixture evenly into 9 tins.
4. Beat egg whites, eggs, grated parmesan cheese, salt and pepper in a medium bowl. Pour into greased tins over broccoli until a little more than 3/4 full. Top with grated cheddar and bake in the oven about 20 minutes or until cooked.
5. Serve immediately.

Peanut Butter & Banana Breakfast Smoothie

SERVINGS: 1
PREP/TOTAL TIME: 5 min.

Ingredients

- 1 cup non-fat milk
- 1 tablespoon all natural peanut butter
- 1 medium banana, frozen or fresh

Instructions

1. Combine all ingredients in food processor or blender. Blend until smooth.

Baked Apple Spice Oatmeal

SERVINGS: 9
PREP TIME: 15 min.
TOTAL TIME: 45 min.

Ingredients

- 1 beaten egg
- 1/2 cup applesauce, sweetened
- 1 1/2 cups non-fat or 1% milk
- 1 teaspoon vanilla
- 2 tablespoons oil
- 1 apple, chopped (about 1 1/2 cups)
- 2 cups rolled oats
- 1 teaspoon baking powder
- 1/4 teaspoon salt
- 1 teaspoon cinnamon
- 2 tablespoons brown sugar
- 2 tablespoons chopped nuts

Instructions

1. Preheat oven to 375°F (190°C). Lightly oil or spray an 8 by 8 inch baking pan.
2. In a bowl, combine egg, applesauce, milk, vanilla, and oil. Add apple
3. In a separate bowl, mix rolled oats, baking powder, salt and cinnamon. Add to the liquid ingredients and combine well. Pour mix into baking dish and bake for 25 minutes.
4. Remove from oven and sprinkle with brown sugar and nuts. Return to oven and broil for 3 to 4 minutes or until top is browned and sugar bubbles.
5. Cut into squares and serve warm.

Strawberry Tapioca

SERVINGS: 4
PREP TIME: 10 min.
TOTAL TIME: 30 min.

Ingredients

- 1/2 cup fresh strawberries, hulled and halved
- 1 1/2 cups water
- 1/4 cup quick-cooking tapioca

Instructions

1. In a food processor or in a blender blend strawberries and water until smooth. Pour into a small saucepan.
2. Add and stir in tapioca. Let stand for 10 minutes or until softened. Bring to a boil over medium heat, stir frequently to prevent sticking. Remove when thick and pour into serving dishes.

Strawberry Salad with Balsamic Vinegar

SERVINGS: 6
PREP TIME: 10 min.
TOTAL TIME: 1 hour 10 min.

Ingredients

- 16 ounce fresh strawberries, hulled and large berries cut in half
- 2 tablespoons balsamic vinegar
- 1/4 cup white sugar
- 1/4 teaspoon freshly ground black pepper, or to taste

Instructions

1. Place strawberries in a bowl and drizzle vinegar over strawberries. Sprinkle with sugar. Stir gently. Cover, and let sit at room temperature for between 1 and 4 hours.
2. Grind pepper over berries before serving.

Blueberry Steel Cut Oat Pancakes with Agave

SERVINGS: 10
PREP/TOTAL TIME: 25 min.

Ingredients

- 1 1/2 cups water
- 1/2 cup steel cut oats
- 1/8 teaspoon sea salt
- 1 cup whole wheat flour
- 1/2 teaspoon baking powder
- 1/2 teaspoon baking soda
- 1 egg
- 1 cup milk
- 1/2 cup Greek yogurt, vanilla flavor
- 1 cup frozen blueberries
- 1/2 cup + 2 tablespoons agave nectar

Instructions

1. Bring water to a boil in a medium pot and add steel cut oats and salt. Reduce heat to a simmer and cook until oats are tender, around 10 minutes. Remove from heat and set aside.
2. Combine whole wheat pastry flour, baking powder and soda, egg, milk and yogurt in a medium mixing bowl. Mix until a batter is formed. Gently fold in blueberries and cooked oats.
3. Heat non-stick skillet over medium heat and coat with cooking spray. Spoon one quarter cup of batter on surface and cook until pancakes are slightly golden, about 2-3 minutes per side.
4. Garnish each pancake with about one tablespoon agave nectar.

LUNCH

Buffalo Chicken Salad Wrap

SERVINGS: 4
PREP TIME: 10 min.
TOTAL TIME: 20 min.

Ingredients

- 3-4 ounces of chicken breasts (can also use leftover or rotisserie chicken).
- 2 whole chipotle peppers
- 1/4 cup white wine vinegar
- 1/4 cup low-calorie mayonnaise
- 2 stalks celery, diced
- 2 carrots, cut into matchsticks
- 1 small yellow onion (about 1/2 cup), diced
- 1/2 cup thinly sliced rutabaga or another root vegetable
- 4 ounces spinach, cut into strips
- 2 whole-grain tortillas (12-inch diameter)

Instructions

1. If using uncooked chicken, preheat oven to 375°F (190°C) or start the grill. Bake or grill chicken breasts for 10 minutes on both sides until interior temperature is 165°F (75°C). Remove, cool and cut the chicken into cubes.
2. Puree chipotle peppers with white wine vinegar and mayonnaise in a blender. In a bowl, place all ingredients except spinach and tortillas. Mix thoroughly.
3. Place 2 ounces of spinach and half the mix in each tortilla and wrap.
4. Cut each in half to serve.

Chicken sliders

SERVINGS: 4
PREP TIME: 10 min.
TOTAL TIME: 1 hour

Ingredients

- 10 ounces ground chicken breast
- 1 tablespoon black pepper
- 1 tablespoon minced garlic
- 1 tablespoon balsamic vinegar
- 1/2 cup minced onion
- 1 fresh chili pepper, minced
- 1 tablespoon fennel seed, crushed
- 4 whole wheat mini buns
- 4 lettuce leaves
- 4 tomato slices

Instructions

1. Combine and mix the first 7 items together. Let set for 1 hour.
2. Form the mix into 2-ounce patties.
3. Grill or broil in the oven until a minimum internal temperature of 165°F (75°C) is reached.
4. Serve on toasted buns with lettuce, tomatoes, and sauce of your choice.

Tuna Melt

SERVINGS: 4
PREP TIME: 10 min.
TOTAL TIME: 20 min.

Ingredients

- 6 ounces white tuna packed in water, drained
- 1/3 cup chopped celery
- 1/4 cup chopped onion
- 1/4 cup low fat Russian or Thousand Island salad dressing
- 2 whole-wheat English muffins, split
- 3 ounces reduced-fat Cheddar cheese, grated
- Salt and black pepper, to taste

Instructions

1. Preheat broiler.
2. Combine tuna, celery, onion and salad dressing. Season with salt and pepper.
3. Toast English muffin halves. Place split-side-up on baking sheet and top with a quarter of tuna mixture. Broil 2-3 minutes or until heated through.
4. Top with cheese and return to broiler until cheese is melted, around 1 minute longer.

Curried Garbanzo Beans and Mustard Greens with Sweet Potatoes

SERVINGS: 4
PREP TIME: 10 min.
TOTAL TIME: 35 min.

Ingredients

- 2 medium sweet potatoes, peeled and sliced thin
- 1 medium onion, cut in half and sliced thin
- 2 medium cloves garlic, sliced
- 1/2 cup + 1 tablespoons low sodium chicken or vegetable broth
- 1/2 teaspoon curry powder
- 1/4 teaspoon turmeric
- 2 cups chopped and rinsed mustard greens
- 1 (15 ounce) can sodium free diced tomatoes
- 1 (15 ounce) can garbanzo beans (chickpeas), drained and rinsed
- 2 tablespoon extra-virgin olive oil
- white pepper, to taste

Instructions

1. Steam sweet potatoes for around 5–8 minutes.
2. Heat 1 tablespoon of broth in large skillet. Sauté onion over medium heat in broth for about 4–5 minutes until translucent, stirring frequently.
3. Add garlic, curry powder, turmeric, and mustard greens. Cook, occasionally stirring until mustard greens are wilted, around 5 minutes. Add garbanzo beans, diced tomatoes, salt and pepper. Cook for another 5 minutes.
4. Mash sweet potatoes with olive oil, salt and pepper.
5. Serve mustard greens with mashed sweet potatoes.

Roasted Brussel Sprouts and Caramelized Butternut Squash with Quinoa

SERVINGS: 6
PREP TIME: 10 min.
TOTAL TIME: 40 min.

Ingredients

- 1 cup quinoa, rinsed
- 2 cups low sodium chicken broth
- 9 ounces shaved Brussels sprouts
- 2 tablespoons extra virgin olive oil, divided
- Garlic powder & pepper, to taste
- 2 cups butternut squash, 1/2 inch cubed
- 1 tablespoon brown sugar
- 1/3 cup grated parmesan cheese

Instructions

1. In a saucepan bring broth to a boil then add rinsed quinoa. Cover then turn heat down to medium-low and simmer about 15 minutes or until tender. Fluff with a fork and set aside.
2. Preheat oven to 375°F (190°C) and line a baking sheet with foil. Add Brussels sprouts, 1 tablespoon oil, garlic powder, and pepper to baking sheet. Toss to evenly coat. Roast 15 minutes or until brown and golden.
3. In a large cast iron or heavy bottomed skillet, heat 1 tablespoon oil over medium-high heat. Add brown sugar and butternut squash. Sauté, stirring occasionally until tender, about 15 minutes.
4. In a large bowl combine quinoa, Brussels sprouts, butternut squash, and parmesan cheese. Toss and serve with extra parmesan cheese, if desired.

Turkey, Pear, and Cheese Sandwich

SERVINGS: 2
PREP/TOTAL TIME: 10 min.

Ingredients

- 2 slices multi-grain or rye sandwich bread
- 2 teaspoon Dijon-style mustard
- 2 slices (1 oz. each) reduced-sodium cooked or smoked turkey
- 1 pear, cored and thinly sliced
- 1/4 cup shredded low fat mozzarella cheese
- Coarsely ground pepper, to taste

Instructions

1. Spread each slice of bread with 1 teaspoon mustard. Place one slice turkey on each slice. Arrange pear slices on turkey. Sprinkle each with 2 tablespoons of cheese and some pepper.
2. Broil for 2 to 3 minutes, 4 to 6 inches from heat, or until turkey and pears are warm and the cheese has melted. Cut each sandwich in half and serve open face.

Salmon Salad Pita

SERVINGS: 2
PREP/TOTAL TIME: 5 min.

Ingredients

- 3/4 cup canned Alaskan salmon
- 3 tablespoons plain fat-free yogurt
- 1 tablespoon lemon juice
- 2 tablespoons red bell pepper, minced
- 1 tablespoon red onion, minced
- 1 teaspoon capers, rinsed and chopped
- Pinch of dill, fresh or dried
- Black pepper to taste
- 3 lettuce leaves
- 3 pieces small whole wheat pita bread

Instructions

1. Mix all ingredients together, except lettuce and pita bread, in a small bowl. Place 1 lettuce leaf and 1/3 cup salmon salad inside each pita.

Turkey Apple Gyro

SERVINGS: 6
PREP/TOTAL TIME: 10 min.

Ingredients

- 1 tablespoon vegetable oil
- 1 cup onion, sliced
- 1 cup sweet red pepper, thinly sliced
- 1 cup sweet green pepper, thinly sliced
- 2 tablespoons lemon juice
- 1/2 pound cooked turkey or chicken breast, cut into thin strips
- 1 Golden Delicious apple, cored and finely chopped
- 6 whole wheat pocket pita bread, warmed
- 1/2 cup low fat or fat free plain yogurt

Instructions

1. Heat oil over medium heat in a large skillet. Add onion, peppers, and lemon juice. Cook until tender.
2. Add turkey and apple and cook until turkey is heated through.
3. Remove from heat.
4. Fill each pita with some of the cooked mix.
5. Drizzle with yogurt and serve warm.

Southwest Style Rice Bowl

SERVINGS: 2
PREP TIME: 20 min.
TOTAL TIME: 30 min.

Ingredients

- 1 teaspoon vegetable oil
- 1 cup chopped vegetables (bell peppers, onion, corn, tomato, zucchini, etc.)
- 1 cup cooked meat or tofu (chopped or shredded)
- 1 cup cooked brown rice
- 4 tablespoons salsa
- 2 tablespoons shredded cheese
- 2 tablespoons low fat sour cream

Instructions

1. Heat oil in a medium sized skillet over medium high heat (or 350°F (175°C) in an electric skillet). Add vegetables and cook for 3 to 5 minutes or until vegetables are tender-crisp.
2. Add cooked meat or tofu and cooked rice to skillet until heated through.
3. Divide rice mix between two bowls. Top with salsa, cheese, sour cream and serve warm.

Sunshine Wrap

SERVINGS: 4
PREP TIME: 10 min.
TOTAL TIME: 15 min.

Ingredients

- 8 ounces chicken breast (one large breast)
- 1/2 cup celery, diced
- 2/3 cup canned mandarin oranges, drained
- 1/4 cup onion, minced
- 2 tablespoons mayonnaise
- 1 teaspoon soy sauce
- 1/4 teaspoon garlic powder
- 1/4 teaspoon black pepper
- 1 large whole wheat tortilla
- 4 large lettuce leaves, washed and patted dry

Instructions

1. In a non-stick pan, cook chicken breast on medium-high heat until cooked throughout (internal temperature of 165°F). When chicken has cooled, cut into 1/2 inch cubes.
2. Mix chicken, celery, oranges and onions in a medium bowl. Add mayonnaise, soy sauce, garlic and pepper. Mix until chicken is evenly coated.
3. Lay tortilla on large plate. With a knife or clean kitchen scissors cut tortilla into four quarters. Place 1 lettuce leaf on each tortilla quarter, trimming it so it doesn't hang over tortilla. Put 1/4 of the chicken mixture in the middle of each lettuce leaf. Roll tortillas into a cone.

Tuna Pita Pockets

SERVINGS: 6
PREP/TOTAL TIME: 10 min.

Ingredients

- 1 1/2 cups shredded romaine lettuce
- 3/4 cup diced tomatoes
- 1/2 cup finely chopped green bell peppers
- 1/2 cup shredded carrots
- 1/2 cup finely chopped broccoli
- 1/4 cup finely chopped onion
- 2 cans (6 ounces each) low-salt white tuna packed in water, drained
- 1/2 cup low-fat ranch dressing
- 3 whole-wheat pita pockets, cut in half

Instructions

1. Add the lettuce, tomatoes, peppers, carrots, broccoli and onions in a large bowl. Toss to mix.
2. Add tuna and ranch dressing in a small bowl. Stir to combine. Combine tuna mix with the lettuce mix.
3. Scoop 3/4 cup of the tuna salad into each pita pocket half and serve.

SALADS

Citrus Salad

SERVINGS: 4
PREP/TOTAL TIME: 15 min.

Ingredients

- 2 oranges
- 1 red grapefruit
- 2 tablespoons orange juice
- 2 tablespoons olive oil
- 1 tablespoon balsamic vinegar
- 4 cups spring greens
- 2 tablespoons pine nuts
- 2 tablespoons chopped mint for garnish (optional)

Instructions

1. Remove white pith and membrane of each orange and grapefruit. For each orange section remove the seeds.
2. In a bowl, combine orange juice, olive oil and vinegar. Pour mix over fruit segments and toss gently to evenly coat.
3. Divide spring greens among individual plates. Top each with the fruit and dressing mix. Sprinkle each with 1/2 tablespoon pine nuts. Garnish with chopped mint (optional).

Raw Kale Salad with Lemon Tahini Dressing

SERVINGS: 4
PREP/TOTAL TIME: 15 min. + refrigeration

Ingredients

Lemon Tahini Dressing:

- Makes about 1 cup of dressing
- Ingredients:
- 3 tablespoons Tahini
- 1 tablespoon fat-free Greek Yogurt
- 2 garlic gloves
- Juice from 2 lemons, about 1/2 cup
- 1 teaspoon pepper
- Pinch of salt
- 3 tablespoons of water, or as needed

Salad:

- 1/2 large head of kale, about 4-6 cups
- 1 cup finely chopped red onion
- 1 cup red bell pepper, chopped
- 1/2 cup carrot, chopped
- 1 cup cherry tomatoes, cut in half
- 1/2 cup cucumber, chopped
- 1/4 cup chopped almonds
- 1/4 cup reduced-fat shredded parmesan

Instructions

1. Add all dressing ingredients to a food processor, and blend until smooth. Set aside.
2. Wash kale under cold water and pat dry. Cut leaves from stems and chop into bite sized pieces. Place in a large bowl.
3. Top kale with chopped vegetables and walnuts. Toss.

4. Pour dressing and combine until all ingredients are covered. Top with cheese. Place in refrigerator and let marinate for about 15 minutes or cover and refrigerate for 24 hours.

Black Bean Southwest Salad

SERVINGS: 13
PREP/TOTAL TIME: 10 min. + refrigeration

Ingredients

- 1 can (15.5 ounce) black beans, rinsed and drained
- 9 ounce cooked corn, fresh or frozen (thawed if frozen)
- 1 medium tomato, chopped
- 1/3 cup red onion, chopped
- 1 scallion, chopped
- 2 limes, juice of
- 1 tablespoon olive oil
- 2 tablespoon fresh minced cilantro
- 1 teaspoon salt
- 1 teaspoon fresh black pepper
- 1/2 medium hass avocado, diced
- 1/4 cup queso fresco (cotija) cheese
- 1 diced jalapeno (optional)

Instructions

1. Combine beans, corn, tomato, onion, scallion, cilantro, salt and pepper in a large bowl. Squeeze fresh lime juice to taste and stir in olive oil. Marinate in the refrigerator 30 minutes.
2. Add avocado and cheese before serving.

Mediterranean Tuna Salad

SERVINGS: 10
PREP/TOTAL TIME: 5 min.

Ingredients

- 3 cans (5 ounces each) tuna in water, drained
- 1 cup shredded carrot
- 2 cups diced cucumber
- 1 1/2 cups peas, canned and drained or thawed from frozen
- 3/4 cup low-fat, low-sodium Italian salad dressing

Instructions

1. Place drained tuna in a medium bowl. Break apart chunks with a fork. Add carrot, cucumber, peas and salad dressing. Mixing well.
2. Serve immediately or cover and refrigerate until ready to serve.

Tangy Mango Salad

SERVINGS: 6
PREP/TOTAL TIME: 10 min.

Ingredients

- 3 ripe mangoes, pitted and cubed
- Juice of 1 lime
- 1 teaspoon minced red onion
- 2 tablespoons chopped fresh cilantro leaves
- Half of 1 jalapeno pepper, seeded and minced

Instructions

1. Combine all ingredients in a mixing bowl and let stand 10 minutes.
2. Toss before serving.

Winter Citrus Salad

SERVINGS: 6
PREP/TOTAL TIME: 10 min.

Ingredients

- 8 cups mixed greens (spinach, arugula, red leaf lettuce)
- 2 ruby red grapefruits, peeled and cut into sections
- 2 navel oranges, peeled and cut into sections
- 1/2 avocado, cubed
- 1/4 cup sliced almonds, toasted
- 2 ounces Asiago cheese, shaved
- 4 tablespoons of your favorite balsamic vinaigrette dressing

Instructions

1. Toss ingredients together in a large salad bowl.
2. Serve.

Pineapple Chicken Salad with Balsamic Vinaigrette

SERVINGS: 8
PREP TIME: 5 min.
TOTAL TIME: 15 min.

Ingredients

- 4 boneless, skinless chicken breasts (5 ounces each)
- 1 tablespoon olive oil
- 1 can (8 ounces) unsweetened pineapple chunks, drained (set aside 2 tablespoons of juice)
- 2 cups broccoli florets
- 4 cups fresh baby spinach leaves
- 1/2 cup thinly sliced red onions
- 1/4 cup olive oil
- 2 tablespoons balsamic vinegar
- 2 teaspoons sugar
- 1/4 teaspoon ground cinnamon

Instructions

1. Cut each chicken breast into cubes. Heat olive oil over medium heat in a large, non-stick frying pan. Add chicken and cook until golden brown, about 10 minutes.
2. In a large serving bowl, combine cooked chicken, pineapple chunks, broccoli, spinach and onions.
3. In a small bowl, whisk together the olive oil, vinegar, reserved pineapple juice, sugar and cinnamon. Pour over the salad and gently toss to coat. Serve immediately.

Grilled Chicken Avocado and Mango Salad

SERVINGS: 4
PREP/TOTAL TIME: 7 min.

Ingredients

- 12 ounce grilled chicken breast, sliced
- 1 cup diced avocado
- 1 cup diced mango
- 2 tablespoons diced red onion
- 6 cups baby red butter lettuce
- 2 tablespoons olive oil
- 2 tablespoons white balsamic vinegar

Instructions

1. Whisk olive oil and balsamic vinegar together. Set aside.
2. Toss together avocado, mango, chicken, and red onion.
3. Fill a large salad platter with baby greens or divide them amongst four plates.
4. Top greens with chicken and avocado mix.
5. Drizzle vinegar dressing among the four servings.

Southwestern Black Bean Cakes with Guacamole

SERVINGS: 4
PREP TIME: 10 min.
TOTAL TIME: 20 min.

Ingredients

- 2 slices whole wheat bread, torn
- 3 tablespoons fresh cilantro
- 2 cloves garlic
- 1 can (15-ounce) low sodium black beans, rinsed and drained
- 1 can (7-ounce) chipotle peppers in adobo sauce
- 1 teaspoon ground cumin
- 1 large egg
- 1/2 medium avocado, seeded and peeled
- 1 tablespoon lime juice
- 1 small plum tomato

Instructions

1. Place torn bread in a blender. Cover and blend until bread turns into coarse crumbs. Transfer to a large bowl and set aside.
2. Process cilantro and garlic until finely chopped. Add beans, 1 of the chipotle peppers, 1 to 2 teaspoons of adobo sauce, and cumin. Process by pulsing in a blender until beans are coarsely chopped and mix pull away from sides.
3. Add mix to bread crumbs in bowl. Add egg and combine well.
4. Shape mixture into four 1/2-inch-thick patties. Grill directly over medium heat for 8 to 10 minutes or until patties are heated through, turning once.
5. To make guacamole, mash avocado in small bowl. Stir in lime juice and season with salt and pepper. Serve patties with guacamole and tomato.

Almond Chicken Pear Salad

SERVINGS: 4
PREP/ TOTAL TIME: 5 min.

Ingredients

- 2 cups cooked boneless, skinless, chicken breasts, cut in 1/2-inch cubes
- 1/2 cup green pepper, sliced lengthwise
- 1/4 cup diced celery
- 1/4 teaspoon salt
- 1/2 cup low-fat plain yogurt
- 2 tablespoons reduced-calorie mayonnaise
- 1/2 teaspoon prepared mustard
- 1/4 teaspoon ground ginger
- 2 fresh Pears, cored and cut in 1-inch cubes
- Favorite lettuce
- 2 tablespoons toasted slivered almonds

Instructions

1. Toss together chicken, green pepper and celery. Sprinkle with salt.
2. Combine yogurt, mayonnaise, mustard and ginger. Add to chicken mixture.
3. Add in the pears to the mixture.
4. Serve on individual lettuce-lined salad plates and sprinkle with almonds.

Curried Garbanzo Beans and Mustard Greens with Sweet Potatoes

SERVINGS: 4
PREP TIME: 10 min.
TOTAL TIME: 35 min.

Ingredients

- 2 medium sweet potatoes, peeled and sliced thin
- 1 medium onion, cut in half and sliced thin
- 2 medium cloves garlic, sliced
- 1/2 cup + 1 tablespoons low sodium vegetable broth
- 1/2 teaspoon curry powder
- 1/4 teaspoon turmeric
- 2 cups chopped and rinsed mustard greens
- 1 (15 ounce) can sodium free diced tomatoes
- 1 (15 ounce) can garbanzo beans (chickpeas), drained and rinsed
- 2 tablespoon extra-virgin olive oil
- white pepper, to taste

Instructions

1. Steam sweet potatoes for around 5–8 minutes.
2. Heat 1 tablespoon of broth in large skillet. Sauté onion over medium heat in broth for about 4–5 minutes until translucent, stirring frequently.
3. Add garlic, curry powder, turmeric, and mustard greens. Cook, occasionally stirring until mustard greens are wilted, around 5 minutes. Add garbanzo beans, diced tomatoes, salt and pepper. Cook for another 5 minutes.
4. Mash sweet potatoes with olive oil, salt and pepper.
5. Serve mustard greens with mashed sweet potatoes.

Mango Curry Chicken Salad

SERVINGS: 4
PREP/TOTAL TIME: 7 min.

Ingredients

- 2 1/2 cups (1/2 inch pieces) grilled skinless, boneless chicken breasts
- 3/4 cup plain, non-fat yogurt
- 1 teaspoon curry
- 1/4 cup cubed mango
- 1 cup dried, sweetened cranberries
- 1/4 cup walnuts, coarsely chopped
- 1/3 cup Mozzarella cheese, cut into small cubes

Instructions

1. In a medium bowl, whisk yogurt and curry together. Stir in chicken, mango, cranberries, walnuts and Mozzarella cheese.
2. Mix well and serve on lettuce leaves, if desired.

Avocado Salad with Ginger-Miso Dressing

SERVINGS: 6
PREP/TOTAL TIME: 15 min. + refrigeration

Ingredients

- 1/3 cup plain silken tofu
- 1/3 cup low-fat plain soy milk (soya milk)
- 1 tablespoon peeled and minced fresh ginger
- 1 1/2 teaspoons reduced-sodium soy sauce
- 1 teaspoon light miso
- 1 teaspoon Dijon mustard
- 1 tablespoon chopped fresh cilantro (fresh coriander)
- 1 tablespoon chopped green (spring) onion, including tender green top
- 1 small avocado, pitted, peeled and cut into 12 thin slices
- 1 tablespoon fresh lemon juice
- 12 ounces mixed baby lettuces
- 1/4 cup chopped red onion
- 1 green (spring) onion, including tender green top, thinly sliced on the diagonal
- 1 tablespoon chopped fresh cilantro (fresh coriander)

Instructions

1. In a blender or food processor add tofu, soy milk, ginger, soy sauce, miso and mustard. Process until smooth and creamy. Transfer to a bowl and stir in the cilantro and green onion. Cover and refrigerate for at least 1 hour.
2. Toss avocado slices in the lemon juice in a small bowl. Set aside.
3. Combine the lettuces, red and green onions, and cilantro in a large bowl. Toss to mix.
4. Add 2/3 of the dressing and toss to coat. Divide salad among individual plates.
5. Arrange 2 avocado slices on top of each portion in a crisscross pattern. Top each avocado cross with a spoonful of remaining dressing. Serve immediately.

Spring Nicoise Potato Salad

SERVINGS: 4
PREP TIME: 10 min.
TOTAL TIME: 20 min.

Ingredients

- 8 small red potatoes
- 1 can (6-ounce) white tuna in water, drained
- 12 steamed asparagus spears
- 8 radishes
- 9 pitted Kalamata olives
- 2 tablespoons minced red onion
- 3 tablespoons red wine vinegar
- 2 tablespoons chopped fresh parsley
- 4 teaspoons olive oil
- Black pepper, to taste

Instructions

1. Wash potatoes and leave skins on. Cut into quarters and place in large pot filled with enough water to cover potatoes. Set heat to high and bring water to boil. Boil potatoes for 10 minutes or until tender. Drain water.
2. Place potatoes on platter with tuna, asparagus, radishes, olives and onion.
3. Whisk vinegar, parsley, and oil in small bowl. Drizzle mix over the salad. Add salt and pepper, to taste.

Strawberries, Blue Cheese, and Chicken Mixed Greens Salad with Poppy Seed Dressing

SERVINGS: 4
PREP TIME: 15 min.
TOTAL TIME: 20 min.

Ingredients

Dressing:

- 1 tablespoon red wine vinegar
- 1 tablespoon cider vinegar
- 2 tablespoons olive oil
- 1 teaspoon minced shallots
- 1 1/2 tablespoon honey
- 1/2 tablespoon poppy seeds

Salad:

- 5 ounces mixed baby greens
- 1/4 cup slivered almonds
- 2 cups sliced strawberries
- 1/4 cup blue cheese
- 12 ounces grilled chicken, sliced

Instructions

1. Place all salad dressing ingredients in a small jar and mix well.
2. Combine all of the salad ingredients in a large bowl.
3. Add dressing to the large bowl and toss salad until the dressing is evenly mixed.
4. Divide evenly among four plates.

Shrimp, Strawberry and Feta Salad

SERVINGS: 4
PREP TIME: 5 min.
TOTAL TIME: 10 min.

Ingredients

- 3 tablespoons extra virgin olive oil
- 2 tablespoons balsamic vinegar
- 2 tablespoons water
- 1/4 teaspoon salt
- 1/4 teaspoon black pepper
- 1/3 cup thinly sliced red onion
- 3/4 pound peeled and deveined raw shrimp
- 2 cups (about 10 ounces) fresh strawberries, stemmed and quartered
- 8 cups mixed salad greens, such as butter lettuce and watercress
- 2 ounces crumbled feta cheese
- 1 small cucumber, sliced (about 24 slices)

Instructions

1. In small bowl, combine olive oil and balsamic vinegar to make vinaigrette.
2. In a large bowl, toss onion with 1 tablespoon of the vinaigrette. Set aside.
3. Grill shrimp for 5 minutes until pink and cooked through, turning once, over a grill or in a pan on stove top.
4. In another small bowl, toss strawberries with 1 tablespoon of the vinaigrette.
5. Toss greens with sliced onions and enough remaining vinaigrette to lightly coat. Divide among 4 chilled salad plates and arrange strawberries and shrimp on top of greens. Sprinkle with cheese and garnish with slices of cucumber, dividing equally.
6. Drizzle any remaining vinaigrette over salad.

Apricot Chicken Pasta Salad

SERVINGS: 4
PREP TIME: 7 min.
TOTAL TIME: 20 min.

Ingredients

Dressing

- 2 apricots cut into quarters
- 2 tablespoons white wine vinegar
- 1/4 teaspoon salt
- 1 tablespoon sugar
- 3 tablespoons olive oil
- 1 tablespoon finely chopped fresh basil

Salad

- 1/4 lb. fusilli (corkscrew) pasta
- 6 fresh apricots cut into quarters
- 2 cups low sodium chicken broth
- 2 skinless, boneless chicken breasts
- 1 red bell pepper cut into long thin strips
- 2 small zucchini ends trimmed, cut in half then into thin strips
- 1 tablespoon chopped fresh basil
- 1 cup apricot basil dressing

Instructions

1. In a blender, combine apricots, white wine vinegar, salt and sugar until well blended. With blender running, slowly add olive oil until thick and smooth. Stir in fresh basil.
2. Bring chicken broth to a boil in a small saucepan. Reduce heat to a simmer and add chicken breasts. Cover pan and continue to simmer until chicken is cooked through, about 6 minutes. Remove chicken from the broth. Allow to cool slightly and shred into bite sized pieces with a fork.
3. Cook pasta according to package directions. Drain and let cool. In a large bowl, combine pasta, apricots, chicken, zucchini, red pepper and basil. Toss lightly with the dressing.

Crispy Citrus Salad with Grilled Cod

SERVINGS: 2
PREP TIME: 5 min.
TOTAL TIME: 15 min.

Ingredients

- 6 ounces baked or broiled cod
- 1 1/2 tablespoons olive oil
- 1 1/2 cups shredded spinach
- 1 1/2 cups shredded kohlrabi
- 1 cup shredded celery
- 1 1/2 cups shredded carrot
- 2 tablespoons shredded fresh basil
- 1 tablespoon minced fresh parsley
- 3/4 cup chopped red bell pepper
- 1 teaspoon black pepper
- 1 tablespoon minced garlic
- Zest and juice of 1 lemon
- Zest and juice of 1 lime
- Zest and juice of 1 orange
- 1 cup grapefruit segments
- 1/2 cup orange segments

Instructions

1. Spray a grill or broiler pan with cooking spray. Turn on grill or preheat broiler.
2. Place cod on grill or broiler pan and brush lightly with oil. Grill or broil 3 to 4 inches from heat until fish flakes easily with a fork, about 10 minutes. If using a food thermometer, fish should reach 145°F (65°C).
3. Toss remaining ingredients together in large bowl, except for grapefruit and orange segments and cod.
4. Divide salad between two plates. Top with cod and citrus pieces.

Cinnamon Pistachio Chicken Salad

SERVINGS: 6
PREP/TOTAL TIME: 5 min.

Ingredients

- 16 ounces cooked boneless, skinless chicken breast
- 1 1/2 cups fat-free plain Greek yogurt
- 1/2 cup pistachios, finely chopped
- 1 teaspoon ground cinnamon
- 1 teaspoon fresh lime juice
- 4 fresh basil leaves, finely chopped
- 1/4 teaspoon ground pepper
- 2 scallions, finely chopped

Instructions

1. Shred cooked chicken breast with a fork. Place in a large mixing bowl.
2. Add remaining ingredients and gently toss to combine.
3. Served chilled or at room temperature.

Rocket and Veggie Ham Salad

SERVINGS: 2
PREP/ TOTAL TIME: 5 min.

Ingredients

- 1 (7 ounce) bag arugula
- 7 ounces of your favorite ham deli slices, torn into thin strips
- 1/4 cup olive oil
- 1/4 cup balsamic vinegar

Instructions

1. Place arugula on a large flat platter.
2. Top with ham.
3. Drizzle olive oil and balsamic vinegar on top.

Soups

Ginger Chicken Noodle Soup

SERVINGS: 8
PREP TIME: 10 min.
TOTAL TIME: 20 min.

Ingredients

- 3 ounces dried soba noodles
- 1 tablespoon olive oil
- 1 large yellow onion, chopped
- 1 tablespoon peeled and minced fresh ginger
- 1 carrot, peeled and finely chopped
- 1 clove garlic, minced
- 4 cups chicken stock or broth
- 2 tablespoons reduced-sodium soy sauce
- 1 pound skinless, boneless chicken breasts, chopped
- 1 cup shelled edamame
- 1 cup plain soy milk
- 1/4 cup chopped fresh cilantro/coriander

Instructions

1. Boil a saucepan 3/4 full of water. Add noodles and cook until tender, about 5 minutes. Drain and set aside.
2. Heat olive oil over medium heat in a large saucepan. Add onion and sauté about 4 minutes or until soft and translucent. Add ginger and carrot and sauté for 1 minute. Add garlic and sauté for 30 seconds, not letting garlic brown. Add in stock and soy sauce and bring to a boil. Add the chicken and edamame. Reduce the heat after boiling to medium-low and simmer until chicken is cooked and the edamame are tender, about 4 minutes. Add soba noodles and soy milk and cook until heated through, without letting it boil.
3. Remove pan from heat and stir in the cilantro. Ladle soup into individual bowls and serve.

Autumn Squash Ginger Bisque

SERVINGS: 5
PREP TIME: 10 min.
TOTAL TIME: 1 hour

Ingredients

- 2 teaspoons vegetable oil
- 2 cups sliced onions
- 2 pounds winter squash, peeled, seeded, and cut into 2-inch cubes (about 4 cups)
- 2 pears, peeled, cored, and diced, or 1 can (15 ounces) sliced pears in juice, drained and chopped
- 2 cloves garlic, peeled and crushed
- 2 tablespoons coarsely chopped, peeled fresh ginger, or 1 teaspoon powdered ginger
- 1/2 teaspoon thyme
- 4 cups low-sodium chicken or vegetable broth
- 1 cup water
- 1 tablespoon lemon juice
- 1/2 cup plain non-fat yogurt

Instructions

1. In a large pot heat oil over medium heat. Add onions and cook for 3 to 4 minutes, stirring constantly until softened. Add squash, pears, garlic, ginger and thyme. Cook for 1 minute while stirring.
2. Add broth and water and bring to a simmer. Reduce heat to low. Cover and simmer 35-45 minutes or until squash is tender.
3. Puree soup in a food processor or blender, in batches if necessary. (Follow manufacturer's directions for pureeing hot liquids if using a blender). Return soup to pot and heat. Stir in lemon juice.
4. Garnish each serving with a dollop of yogurt.

Potato Soup with Brie Cheese and Apple

SERVINGS: 8
PREP TIME: 15 min.
TOTAL TIME: 1 hour

Ingredients

- 1 cup chopped yellow onion
- 1/4 cup sliced leeks (whites only)
- 4 large Granny Smith apples, cored, peeled and quartered
- 1 Granny Smith apple, cored and sliced thinly, for garnish
- 2 cups low-sodium chicken broth
- 1 bay leaf
- 1/4 teaspoon dried thyme
- 3 cups fat-free evaporated milk
- 6 small potatoes, peeled and sliced
- 4 ounces brie cheese, cut into small cubes

Instructions

1. Spray a soup pot with cooking spray. Add onion, leeks and 4 apples. Sauté 5 to 7 minutes over medium heat until softened. Add broth, bay leaf, and thyme. Bring to a boil, reduce heat to low and simmer for 15 minutes. Remove bay leaf. Turn off heat and set the mix aside.
2. While the broth mix is cooking, combine evaporated milk and potatoes in a separate saucepan. Cook over medium heat 15 to 20 minutes until potatoes are tender. Stir frequently. Pour potato mix into soup pot. Stir to evenly mix.
3. In a blender or food processor, puree the soup in batches until smooth, adding pieces of brie cheese during pureeing. Return pureed batch to the soup pot and heat until heated through.
4. Ladle into individual bowls and garnish with thin slices of apple.

Greek Lentil Soup

SERVINGS: 4
PREP TIME: 20 min.
TOTAL TIME: 1 hour 20 min

Ingredients

- 8 ounces brown lentils
- 1/4 cup olive oil
- 1 tablespoon minced garlic
- 1 onion, minced
- 1 large carrot, chopped
- 1 quart water
- 1 pinch dried oregano
- 1 pinch crushed dried rosemary
- 2 bay leaves
- 1 tablespoon tomato paste
- salt and ground black pepper, to taste
- 1 teaspoon olive oil, or to taste
- 1 teaspoon red wine vinegar, to taste

Instructions

1. Place lentils in a large saucepan. Add enough water to cover lentils by an inch. Bring water to a boil and cook about 10 minutes or until tender. Drain.
2. Heat olive oil in a saucepan over medium heat. Add garlic, onion, and carrot. Cook and stir about 5 minutes or until the onion has softened and turned translucent. Pour in lentils, 1 quart water, oregano, rosemary, and bay leaves. Bring to a boil and then reduce heat to medium-low. Cover and simmer for 10 minutes.
3. Stir in tomato paste and season with salt and pepper. Cover and simmer 30 to 40 minutes or until the lentils have softened, occasionally stirring. Add additional water if the soup becomes too thick. Drizzle with 1 teaspoon olive oil and red wine vinegar to taste.

Leftover Turkey Chili

SERVINGS: 6
PREP TIME: 10 min.
TOTAL TIME: 25 min.

Ingredients

- 1 tablespoon olive oil
- 2 tablespoons diced onion
- 2 teaspoon diced garlic
- 1 can (15 ounce) low sodium black beans
- 1 cup shredded precooked white meat turkey
- 3 tablespoons roasted red pepper, canned in water, drained
- 1 can (32 ounces) roasted diced tomato with juice
- 1/2 tablespoon chili powder
- 1 tablespoon cumin
- 1/2 teaspoon red pepper flakes
- 1/2 teaspoon salt
- 6 tablespoons plain fat-free yogurt
- 6 tablespoon shredded cheddar cheese

Instructions

1. Heat oil over medium heat in a large pot. Add onions and garlic and sauté about 3-4 minutes, or until onions are translucent. Add remaining ingredients, except yogurt and cheese and stir thoroughly to combine.
2. Bring chili to a simmer. Cover and let cook for 10-15 minutes.
3. Once chili is done, remove from heat.
4. Serve topped with 1 tablespoon yogurt and 1 tablespoon shredded cheddar cheese.

Roasted Pear and Squash Soup

SERVINGS: 6
PREP TIME: 15 min.
TOTAL TIME: 1 hour

Ingredients

- 2 pounds Delicata Squash or Butternut Squash, cut in half lengthwise and seeded
- 2 tablespoons olive oil
- 2 firm but ripe Anjou or Bartlett pears, cut in half lengthwise and cored
- 4 cups canned low-sodium chicken broth
- 1/4 teaspoon freshly grated nutmeg
- 1 tablespoon sugar
- 1/4 teaspoon pepper
- 1/2 cup fat free evaporated milk

Instructions

1. Preheat the oven to 350°F (175°C).
2. Brush flesh of the squash and pears with olive oil. Place cut side down on a rimmed baking sheet. Place in preheated oven and roast about 30 to 35 minutes or until tender when pierced with a fork.
3. Use a spoon to scrape out the flesh of the squash and pears and place in a blender. Discard skins. Add 1 to 2 cups of the chicken broth and blend until smooth.
4. Place mixture in a 3 1/2-to 4-quart saucepan. Add remaining chicken broth, nutmeg, sugar, and pepper.
5. Bring to a boil, and then reduce to a simmer. Cook for 10 minutes. Stir in the evaporated milk and simmer until just heated through.

Curried Carrot Soup

SERVINGS: 6
PREP TIME: 10 min.
TOTAL TIME: 25 min.

Ingredients

- 1 tablespoon olive oil
- 1 teaspoon mustard seed
- 1/2 yellow onion, chopped
- 1 pound carrots, peeled and cut into 1/2-inch pieces
- 1 tablespoon plus 1 teaspoon peeled and chopped fresh ginger
- 1/2 jalapeno chili, seeded
- 2 teaspoons curry powder
- 5 cups chicken stock, vegetable stock or broth
- 1/4 cup chopped fresh cilantro (fresh coriander), plus leaves for garnish
- 2 tablespoons fresh lime juice
- 1/2 teaspoon salt (optional)
- 3 tablespoons low-fat sour cream or fat-free plain yogurt
- Grated zest of 1 lime

Instructions

1. Heat olive oil over medium heat in a large saucepan. Add the mustard seed. When seeds begin to pop (about 1 minute) add onion and sauté about 4 minutes or until soft and translucent. Add carrots, ginger, jalapeno and curry powder and sauté about 3 minutes or until seasonings are fragrant.
2. Add 3 cups of the stock and raise heat to high. Bring to a boil. Reduce heat to medium-low and simmer about 6 minutes or until carrots are tender.
3. Puree soup in batches in a blender or food processor until smooth. Return to the saucepan. Stir in remaining 2 cups stock. Return soup to medium heat and reheat.
4. Just before serving, stir in chopped cilantro and lime juice. Season with the salt, if desired.
5. Garnish with a drizzle of yogurt, a sprinkle of lime zest and cilantro leaves.

Wild Rice Mushroom Soup

SERVINGS: 4
PREP TIME: 10 min.
TOTAL TIME: 35 min.

Ingredients

- 1 tablespoon olive oil
- half a white onion, chopped
- 1/4 cup chopped celery
- 1/4 cup chopped carrots
- 1 1/2 cups sliced fresh white mushrooms
- 1/2 cup white wine, or 1/2 cup low-sodium, fat-free chicken broth
- 2 1/2 cups low-sodium, fat-free chicken broth
- 1 cup fat-free half-and-half
- 2 tablespoons flour
- 1/4 teaspoon dried thyme
- black pepper
- 1 cup cooked wild rice

Instructions

1. Heat olive oil in pot on medium heat. Add chopped onion, celery and carrots. Cook until tender. Add mushrooms, white wine and chicken broth. Cover until heated through.
2. Blend half-and-half, flour, thyme and pepper in a bowl. Stir in cooked wild rice. Pour rice mix into hot pot with vegetables. Cook over medium heat. Stir continually until bubbly and thickened.
3. Serve warm.

Seafood Chowder

SERVINGS: 6
PREP TIME: 10 min.
TOTAL TIME: 40 min.

Ingredients

- 2 medium potatoes, cubed
- 1 carrot, sliced 1/4 inch thick
- 1 medium onion, chopped
- 1 cup clam juice
- 1 cup water
- 1 tablespoon butter
- 1/4 teaspoon salt
- 1/4 teaspoon pepper
- 1 pound lean fish (halibut, cod, or salmon) cut into 1-inch pieces
- 1 can (6 1/2 ounce) clams, un-drained
- 1 can (12 ounce) evaporated skim milk
- 2 tablespoons chopped fresh chives
- 1 teaspoon paprika

Instructions

1. Combine potatoes, carrots, onion, clam juice, water, butter, salt and pepper in a large saucepan. Bring to a boil. Reduce heat, cover, and simmer 15-20 minutes or until potatoes are almost tender.
2. Stir in fish and clams, and increase heat until soup begins to boil. Reduce heat and simmer 5 minutes or until fish flakes easily with a fork.
3. Stir in milk, chives, and paprika and heat through.
4. Serve.

Spicy Chili Soup

SERVINGS: 8
PREP TIME: 10 min.
TOTAL TIME: 35 min.

Ingredients

- 2 tablespoons olive oil
- 1 pound boneless skinless chicken breast, cubed
- 1 heaping tablespoon garlic, minced
- 1 medium onion, diced
- 1 bell pepper, diced
- 2 large carrots, sliced
- 1/3 cup chili powder
- 1 15 oz. can reduced sodium kidney beans, with liquid
- 2 cans no salt added diced tomatoes, with juice
- 2 cans 50% reduced sodium chicken or beef broth
- Pepper, to taste
- 1/4 teaspoon salt (optional)

Instructions

1. Sauté the cubed chicken breast in the olive oil over medium heat in a large pot, until the chicken has browned on both sides. Remove the chicken and set aside.
2. In the same pot, add in garlic, onion, bell pepper, and carrots. Sauté about 5 minutes until lightly browned, stirring occasionally. Add chili powder to the vegetable mix and sauté another 2-3 minutes.
3. Add the kidney beans with liquid, diced tomatoes with juice, broth, and cooked chicken. Bring the liquid to a simmer for 10-15 minutes or until vegetables are soft.
4. Add salt and pepper if desired. Serve hot.

Shamrock Soup

SERVINGS: 4
PREP TIME: 15 min.
TOTAL TIME: 45 min.

Ingredients

- 1/2 cup each: chopped onion, carrot and celery
- 1 tablespoon butter
- 3/4 cup dry split peas, rinsed and drained
- 1 can (13 3/4 ounces) chicken broth
- 1 1/2 cups fat free milk, divided
- 4 cups washed and dried fresh spinach leaves
- 4 tablespoons diced fully cooked lean ham
- Salt and freshly ground pepper to taste
- Pinch of freshly grated or ground nutmeg

Instructions

1. In a medium saucepan, sauté onion, carrot and celery in butter until onion is soft. Add split peas, chicken broth and half of milk. Bring to a boil, cover and reduce heat to low. Simmer for 30 minutes, occasionally stirring, until split peas are tender. Remove from heat and cool slightly.
2. Puree split pea mixture with spinach in blender or food processor. Return mix to saucepan. Stir in remaining milk until desired consistency. Cook and stir over low heat until mix comes to a simmer. Season to taste with freshly ground pepper and nutmeg.
3. Serve and sprinkle with ham.

Steamy Salmon Chowder

SERVINGS: 8
PREP TIME: 10 min.
TOTAL TIME: 30 min.

Ingredients

- 1 teaspoon olive oil
- 1/2 cup chopped celery
- 1 clove garlic, minced
- 1 can (15-ounce) reduced-sodium chicken broth
- 2 1/2 cups frozen country-style hash browns with green pepper and onion
- 1 cup frozen peas and carrots
- 1/2 teaspoon dill
- 1/2 teaspoon ground pepper
- 6 ounces pouched or canned pink salmon, with bones removed
- 1 can (12-ounce) evaporated skim milk
- 1 can (14 3/4 ounces) no-salt-added, cream-style corn

Instructions

1. In a large saucepan over medium heat, sauté olive oil and celery for 10 minutes. Add garlic and sauté another minute.
2. Add the chicken broth, hash browns, peas and carrots, dill and pepper and bring to a boil. Reduce heat and simmer for about 10 minutes, until the vegetables are cooked.
3. Add salmon, separating into pieces with a fork. Stir in evaporated milk and corn and cook until heated through.

DINNER

Grilled Pineapple Salsa Beef Kabobs

SERVINGS: 6
PREP TIME: 15 min.
TOTAL TIME: 30 min. + margination

Ingredients

- 1-1/2 pounds beef shoulder center (Ranch) steaks, cut 1 inch thick
- Salt and pepper

Marinade:
- 2 tablespoons fresh lime juice
- 2 tablespoons olive oil
- 2 large cloves garlic, minced
- 1 medium jalapeno pepper, minced
- 1/2 teaspoon ground cumin

Pineapple Salsa:
- 1/2 medium pineapple (about 3 cups), peeled, cored, cut into 1-1/2 inch chunks
- 1 medium red onion, cut into 12 wedges
- 1 large red or green bell pepper, cut into 1-1/2 inch pieces
- 2 teaspoons freshly grated lime peel
- 1/2 teaspoon salt

Instructions

1. Cut beef steaks in 1-1/4-inch pieces. In a medium bowl, combine marinade ingredients. Reserve 2 tablespoons of marinade for salsa. Add beef to remaining marinade and toss to coat. Cover and marinate 30 minutes to 2 hours in refrigerator.
2. Remove beef from marinade. Place beef pieces onto six 10-inch metal skewers, leaving small space between pieces, or place fruit and vegetable pieces evenly on six 10-inch metal skewers.

3. Place fruit and vegetable kabobs on a grill over medium, ash-covered coals. Grill uncovered for 12 to 15 minutes, until vegetables are tender, occasionally turn. Remove and keep warm. Place beef kabobs in the center of grid. Grill covered, for 7 to 9 minutes until medium rare to medium doneness, occasionally turning.
4. Remove fruit and vegetables from skewers and coarsely chop. In a medium bowl, combine with reserved marinade, lime peel, and 1/2 teaspoon salt.
5. Season beef with salt and pepper, as desired. Serve with Pineapple Salsa.

Sesame-Honey Chicken and Quinoa

SERVINGS: 4
PREP TIME: 10 min.
TOTAL TIME: 35 min.

Ingredients

- 1 1/2 cups water
- 3/4 cup quinoa, rinsed
- 2 cups grated carrots (about 3 large sized)
- 2 tablespoons rice vinegar
- 2 tablespoons sesame seeds, toasted
- 1 tablespoon sesame oil
- 2 tablespoons sesame oil
- 2 cups cooked chicken breast, cut into bite-sized pieces
- 3 tablespoons honey
- 3 tablespoons reduced-sodium soy sauce
- 2 tablespoons water
- 1 teaspoon corn-starch
- 2 scallions, sliced

Instructions

1. Bring 1 1/2 cups water to a boil in a small saucepan. Add quinoa and return to a boil. Reduce to a simmer, cover and cook until the water is absorbed, around 10 to 14 minutes. Uncover and let stand.
2. In a medium bowl, combine carrots, rice vinegar, sesame seeds, and 1 tablespoon oil. Set aside.
3. In a small bowl, combine sesame oil, honey, soy sauce, 2 tablespoons water and corn-starch. Pour into a medium skillet. Cook over medium heat, and stir until sauce has thickened. Add chicken and stir until coated with sauce, about 1 minute.
4. Divide quinoa among 4 bowls and top each with 1/2 cup carrot slaw and 3/4 cup chicken mix. Sprinkle with scallions.

Shrimp Pasta Primavera

SERVINGS: 6
PREP TIME: 10 min.
TOTAL TIME: 30 min.

Ingredients

- 1-1/4 cup fresh asparagus, sliced into 1 inch lengths (about 1/2 pound)
- 12 ounces whole wheat penne pasta
- 1 cup green peas, fresh or frozen
- 2 teaspoon olive oil
- 1 tablespoon garlic, minced
- 1/8 teaspoon crushed red pepper
- 1 pound medium shrimp, peeled and deveined
- 1/2 cup green onion, thinly sliced
- 2 teaspoon fresh lemon juice
- 1 tablespoon fresh parsley, chopped
- 1/3 cup grated Parmesan cheese
- 1/2 teaspoon salt
- Fresh ground black pepper

Instructions

1. Boil a 6 quart pot of water. Add asparagus and cook until tender-crisp, around 4 minutes. Transfer to a bowl. Add pasta and cook according to the package directions. In the last 2 minutes of cooking, add peas. Drain pasta with the peas and reserve in the bowl with the asparagus.
2. Heat olive oil over medium heat in a 12-inch non-stick skillet. Add minced garlic and crushed red pepper. Cook and stir until fragrant, about 1 minute. Add shrimp and cook for 2 minutes on each side. Add pasta with the vegetables, green onion, lemon juice, parsley and Parmesan cheese. Toss to coat and season with salt and fresh ground black pepper, to taste.

Chicken Pesto Bake

SERVINGS: 4
PREP TIME: 5 min.
TOTAL TIME: 25 min.

Ingredients

- 2 boneless, skinless chicken breasts (160 total ounces)
- 4 teaspoons basil pesto
- 1 medium tomato, sliced thin
- 6 tablespoons shredded reduced fat mozzarella cheese
- 2 teaspoons grated parmesan cheese

Instructions

1. Wash chicken and pat dry with paper towel. Slice chicken breast horizontally to create 4 thin pieces.
2. Preheat the oven to 400°F (200°C). Line a baking sheet with foil or parchment.
3. Place chicken on the baking sheet and spread 1 teaspoon of pesto on chicken piece.
4. Bake until chicken is no longer pink in the center, about 15 minutes. Remove from oven and top with tomatoes, mozzarella, and parmesan cheese.
5. Return to oven for another 3 to 5 minutes or until the cheese melts.

Grilled Chicken with Crunchy Apple Salsa

SERVINGS: 4
PREP TIME: 15 min.
TOTAL TIME: 35 min. + refrigeration

Ingredients

- 2 cups chopped, cored Gala apples
- 1 Anaheim chili pepper, seeded and chopped
- 1/2 cup chopped onion
- 1/4 cup lime juice
- salt and black pepper
- 1/4 cup dry white wine
- 1/4 cup apple juice
- 1/2 teaspoon grated lime zest
- 1/2 teaspoon salt
- 1/8 teaspoon black pepper
- 2 whole boneless, skinless chicken breasts

Instructions

1. In medium bowl, combine apples, chili pepper, onion, lime juice and salt and pepper to taste. Cover and set salsa aside while preparing chicken. You can refrigerate if making a day ahead of time.
2. In a large bowl, combine white wine, apple juice, lime zest, salt, and pepper. Cut chicken breasts in half for a total of four pieces. Add chicken and coat with mixture. Cover and refrigerate for at least half an hour.
3. Drain and discard chicken marinade.
4. Heat grill. Grill chicken until cooked through.
5. Serve with the salsa.

Curried Pork in Apple Cider

SERVINGS: 6
PREP TIME: 15 min.
TOTAL TIME: 45 min.

Ingredients

- 16 ounces pork tenderloin, cut into 6 pieces
- 1 1/2 tablespoons curry powder
- 1 tablespoon extra-virgin olive oil
- 2 medium yellow onions (about 2 cups), chopped
- 2 cups apple cider, divided
- 1 tart apple, peeled, seeded and chopped into chunks
- 1 tablespoon corn-starch

Instructions

1. Season pork tenderloin with curry powder. Let stand for 15 minutes.
2. Heat olive oil over medium-high heat in a large skillet. Add tenderloin and cook, turning once, until browned on both sides, around 5 to 10 minutes. Remove meat from skillet and set aside.
3. Add onions to skillet and sauté until golden and soft. Add 1 1/2 cups of the apple cider, reduce heat and simmer until the liquid is half gone.
4. Add chopped apple, corn-starch and remaining 1/2 cup apple cider. Simmer and stir while sauce thickens, about 2 minutes. Return tenderloin to skillet and simmer for the 5 minutes.
5. Pour thickened sauce over meat and serve immediately.

Halibut with Tomato and Basil Salsa

SERVINGS: 4
PREP TIME: 10 min.
TOTAL TIME: 25 min.

Ingredients

- 2 tomatoes, diced
- 2 tablespoons fresh basil, chopped
- 1 teaspoon fresh oregano, chopped
- 1 tablespoon minced garlic
- 2 teaspoons extra-virgin olive oil
- 4 halibut fillets, each 4 ounces

Instructions

1. Preheat oven to 350°F (175°C).
2. Lightly coat a 9-by-13-inch baking pan with cooking spray.
3. In a small bowl, combine tomato, basil, oregano and garlic. Add olive oil and mix well.
4. Arrange halibut fillets in the baking pan. Spoon tomato mixture on top of the fish.
5. Place in oven and bake until fish is opaque in the middle when tested with the tip of a knife, around 10 to 15 minutes.
6. Transfer individual plates and serve immediately.

Cranberry Chicken

SERVINGS: 4
PREP TIME: 5 min.
TOTAL TIME: 20 min.

Ingredients

- 1 pound boneless, skinless chicken breasts
- 1 teaspoon butter
- 1/4 teaspoon black pepper
- 3/4 cup whole cranberry sauce
- 1/4 cup chili sauce
- 1/4 cup apple juice
- 1 teaspoon brown sugar

Instructions

1. Sprinkle chicken with pepper. Pound the meat.
2. In a large pan, brown the chicken in butter.
3. Add remaining ingredients and simmer for 15 minutes, covered.
4. Remove lid and boil until sauce is desired thickness.

Whiskey-Mushroom New York Strip Steak

SERVINGS: 2
PREP TIME: 10 min.
TOTAL TIME: 35 min.

Ingredients

- 2 New York strip steaks (4 ounces each) trimmed of all visible fat
- 1 teaspoon margarine
- 3 garlic cloves, chopped
- 2 ounces sliced shiitake mushrooms
- 2 ounces button mushrooms
- 1/4 teaspoon thyme
- 1/4 teaspoon rosemary
- 1/4 cup whiskey

Instructions

1. Lightly coat grill rack or broiler pan with cooking spray and place cooking rack 4 to 6 inches from the heat source.
2. Preheat a gas grill or broiler.
3. Grill or broil the steaks, about 10 minutes on each side, until slightly pink on the inside, or until a food thermometer indicates 145°F (65°C), 160°F (70°C) (medium) or 170°F (75°C) (well done). Transfer to a plate and keep warm.
4. In a small saucepan, heat the margarine over medium heat. Add garlic, mushrooms, thyme and rosemary. Sauté until the mushrooms are tender, about 1 to 2 minutes. Remove and carefully add the whiskey (be careful of flame). Stir sauce for another minute.
5. Top steaks with mushrooms sauce and immediately serve.

Pear Curry Chicken

SERVINGS: 6
PREP TIME: 10 min.
TOTAL TIME: 30 min.

Ingredients

- 2 ripe pears, divided
- 1 tablespoon vegetable oil
- 1 cup diced onion
- 1 tablespoon curry powder
- 1 teaspoon minced garlic
- 1 teaspoon salt
- 3/4 teaspoon ground ginger
- 3/4 teaspoon ground cinnamon
- 1/4 teaspoon ground black pepper
- 3 chicken breasts (1 1/2 pounds), halved, boneless, skinless, cut into 1-inch cubes
- 1 can (14 ounces) light coconut milk
- 1/3 cup raisins (optional)

Instructions

1. Peel and core 1 pear. Puree and set aside.
2. Heat oil over medium heat in large frying pan. Add onion, curry powder, garlic, salt, ginger, cinnamon, and pepper and sauté 5 minutes, occasionally stirring, until onions are transparent.
3. Add chicken, and continue to sauté 5 minutes, stirring occasionally, until browned. A
4. Add pureed pear, coconut milk, and raisins. Simmer for 5 minutes.
5. Core and cut remaining pear into 1/2-inch cubes and add to curry. Simmer for 5 minutes and serve.

Mustard-Dill Poached Salmon

SERVINGS: 4
PREP TIME: 10 min.
TOTAL TIME: 30 min.

Ingredients

- 1 teaspoon olive or vegetable oil
- 2 tablespoon shallots, finely chopped
- 1 1/2 cup fat-free or low-fat milk
- 1/2 teaspoon salt
- Freshly ground black pepper to taste
- 1 1/4 pounds salmon fillet, about 1 inch thick, skin on, cut into 4 portions
- 1 tablespoons fresh lemon juice
- 1 1/2 teaspoons corn-starch
- 2 tablespoons chopped fresh dill
- 1/4 cup reduced-fat sour cream
- 2 teaspoons Dijon mustard
- Lemon wedges and fresh dill sprigs, for garnish

Instructions

1. Heat oil over medium heat in a large skillet or sauté pan. Add shallots and sauté until softened, about 30 to 60 seconds. Add milk, shallots, salt and pepper. Bring to simmer while stirring. Reduce heat to low.
2. Place salmon pieces in milk sauce, skin-side up, and immediately turn over. Cover and gently poach salmon, occasionally spooning milk liquid over top of salmon, about 10 to 12 minutes or just until interior is opaque.
3. Carefully transfer salmon to a warm platter. Cover with foil and keep warm.
4. In a small bowl, mix lemon juice and corn-starch. Add mix to poaching liquid and cook, constantly stirring, until slightly thickened, about 1 minute. Stir in sour cream, chopped dill and mustard.
5. Garnish salmon with lemon wedges and dill sprigs. Serve with the mustard-dill sauce.

Fish Cod Fillet Tacos

SERVINGS: 8
PREP TIME: 15 min.
TOTAL TIME: 35 min.

Ingredients

Fish

- 2 pounds cod fillets
- 3 tablespoons lime juice (or juice from 2 limes)
- 1 tomato, chopped
- 1/2 onion, chopped
- 3 tablespoons cilantro, chopped
- 1 teaspoon olive oil
- 1/4 teaspoon cayenne pepper (optional)
- 1/4 teaspoon black pepper
- 1/4 teaspoon salt

Slaw

- 2 cups red cabbage, shredded
- 1/2 cup green onions, chopped
- 3/4 cup non-fat sour cream
- 3/4 cup salsa
- 8 6-inch corn tortillas

Instructions

1. Preheat oven to 350°F (175°C).
2. Rinse fish and drain fat off by placing on rack in baking dish.
3. Combine lime juice, tomato, onion, cilantro, olive oil, peppers, and salt and spoon on top of fillets. Keep fish moist by covering loosely with aluminium foil. Bake 15-20 minutes or until fish flakes.
4. Mix cabbage and onion.
5. Combine sour cream and salsa and add to cabbage mixture.
6. Divide fish among tortillas. Add 1/4 cup of slaw to each.

Garlic and Lime Pork Chops

SERVINGS: 4
PREP TIME: 20 min.
TOTAL TIME: 35 min.

Ingredients

- 4 (6 ounces each) lean boneless pork chops
- 4 cloves garlic, crushed
- 1 teaspoon cumin
- 1 teaspoon chili powder
- 1 teaspoon paprika
- Fresh black pepper to taste
- 1 tablespoon of lime juice (about 1/2 lime)
- Zest of 1/2 lime (about 1 teaspoon)

Instructions

1. Trim fat off pork.
2. In a large bowl season pork with garlic, cumin, chili powder, paprika, and pepper. Add lime juice and lime zest. Allow pork to marinate for at least 20 minutes.
3. Line a broiler pan with foil. Place pork chops on the broiler pan and broil for around 4-5 minutes on each side, or until browned.

Honey Crusted Chicken

SERVINGS: 2
PREP TIME: 10 min.
TOTAL TIME: 35 min.

Ingredients

- 8 saltine crackers, each about 2 inches
- 1 teaspoon paprika
- 2 boneless, skinless chicken breasts (4 ounces each)
- 4 teaspoons honey

Instructions

1. Preheat oven to 375°F (190°C). Lightly coat baking dish with cooking spray.
2. Crush crackers and place in a small bowl. Add paprika and mix well.
3. Add chicken and honey in a separate bowl. Toss to evenly coat. Add cracker mixture and press chicken in until it's evenly coated on both sides.
4. Place chicken in the prepared baking dish. Bake until lightly browned and cooked through, about 20 to 25 minutes. Serve immediately.

Spicy Mango Jerk Chicken

SERVINGS: 4
PREP TIME: 20 min
TOTAL TIME: 45 min

Ingredients

- 2 ripe mangos, peeled, pitted and cut into 1/4-inches
- 1/4 cup lime juice
- 2 tablespoon brown sugar
- 1/2 teaspoon crushed red pepper
- 1/4 teaspoon garlic powder
- 1/4 teaspoon cinnamon
- 1/4 teaspoon ground allspice
- 4 boneless, skinless chicken breasts, slightly flattened (about 1 1/2 pounds)
- 2 tablespoon Jamaican jerk seasoning blend
- 1 lime, halved

Instructions

1. In a medium bowl, combine mango, lime juice, brown sugar, red pepper, garlic powder, cinnamon and allspice. Set aside.
2. Rinse chicken and pat dry. Sprinkle both sides with jerk seasoning and let stand for 10 minutes.
3. Cook on a well-oiled grill over medium heat for about 5 to 7 minutes on each side, or until chicken is cooked through. Remove and squeeze lime halves over chicken.
4. Top with spicy mango mixture.

Lemon Chicken and Potatoes

SERVINGS: 4
PREP TIME: 10 min.
TOTAL TIME: 45 min.

Ingredients

- 1 1/2 pounds boneless skinless chicken breasts, cut into 1-inch cubes
- 1 pound Yukon Gold potatoes, cut into 3/4-inch cubes
- 1 medium onion, coarsely chopped
- 1/2 cup reduced-fat Greek or olive oil vinaigrette
- 1/4 cup lemon juice
- 1 teaspoon dry oregano
- 1 teaspoon minced garlic
- 1/2 cup chopped tomato

Instructions

1. In a large bowl, mix all ingredients except tomatoes. Place equal amounts on 4 large squares of heavy-duty aluminium foil. Enclose and fold sides of each to enclose filling. Leave room to allow air to circulate.
2. Grill over medium heat for 25 to 30 minutes or until chicken is cooked through and potatoes are soft.
3. Carefully open each foil and sprinkle equal amounts of tomato.

Pork Medallions with Herbes de Provence

SERVINGS: 2
PREP TIME: 10 min.
TOTAL TIME: 25 min.

Ingredients

- 8 ounces pork tenderloin, trimmed of visible fat and cut crosswise into 6 pieces
- Freshly ground black pepper, to taste
- 1/2 teaspoon herbes de Provence
- 1/4 cup dry white wine

Instructions

1. Sprinkle pork with black pepper. Place pork between sheets of wax paper and pound with a mallet or roll with a rolling pin until about 1/4-inch thick.
2. In a large, non-stick frying pan, cook the pork over medium-high heat, about 2 to 3 minutes on each side. Remove from heat and sprinkle with herbes de Provence. Place the pork on individual plates and keep warm.
3. Pour wine into frying pan and cook until boiling. Scrape brown bits from the bottom of the pan. Pour the wine sauce over the pork and serve immediately.

Pork Tenderloin with Apples and Balsamic Vinegar

SERVINGS: 4
PREP TIME: 10 min.
TOTAL TIME: 35 min.

Ingredients

- 1 tablespoon olive oil
- 1 pound pork tenderloin, trimmed of all visible fat
- Freshly ground black pepper, to taste
- 2 cups chopped onion
- 2 cups chopped apple
- 1 1/2 tablespoons fresh rosemary, chopped
- 1 cup low-sodium chicken broth
- 1 1/2 tablespoons balsamic vinegar

Instructions

1. Preheat oven to 450°F (230°C). Lightly coat a baking pan with cooking spray.
2. In a large skillet, heat olive oil over high heat. Add pork and sprinkle with black pepper. Cook until browned on all sides, about 3 minutes. Remove from heat and place in the prepared baking pan. Roast the pork for 15 minutes, or until a food thermometer reads 165°F (75°C) (medium).
3. Add onion, apple and rosemary to the skillet. Sauté over medium heat, about 3 to 5 minutes or until onions and apples are soft. Stir in the broth and vinegar. Increase heat and boil until the sauce is reduced, about 5 minutes.
4. Place pork on a large platter. Slice on the diagonal and put on 4 warmed plates. Scoop onion-apple sauce over top and serve immediately.

Salsa Verde Burger

SERVINGS: 4
PREP TIME: 15 min.
TOTAL TIME: 45 min.

Ingredients

- 2 tomatillos
- 1 serrano chile pepper, sliced
- 1/4 cup onion, sliced
- 1/4 teaspoon chopped garlic
- 1 teaspoon black pepper
- 4 (93% lean) beef patties (4.75 ounces each)
- 1/2 cup salsa verde
- 4 slices reduced-fat pepper jack cheese
- 4 whole-wheat hamburger buns
- 1/4 cup shredded red cabbage
- 4 ounces sliced avocado

Instructions

1. Place the tomatillos, Serrano peppers, onion, and garlic in a saucepan. Just cover with water and bring to a boil. Reduce heat to medium-low and cook until the tomatillos are soft and are slightly brown, about 20-30 minutes. Add more water if needed to keep from burning.
2. Pour cooked vegetables into a blender and blend until smooth.
3. Heat a skillet or grill over high heat.
4. When hot, spray with cooking spray or lightly oil. Add the patties.
5. Season with pepper and cook a few minutes on each side, as desired.
6. Add cheese and cover. Cook to melt, about 30 seconds.
7. Place the cooked burgers on the buns and top each with 2 tablespoons salsa verde, red cabbage, and avocado slices.

Brazilian Black Beans Sausage

SERVINGS: 8
PREP TIME: 15 min.
TOTAL TIME: 50 min.

Ingredients

- 2 teaspoons vegetable oil
- 8 ounces low-fat polish kielbasa sausage, cut into small pieces
- 1 large onion, chopped
- 1/8 teaspoon garlic powder or 1 clove garlic, minced
- 1 red bell pepper, chopped
- 1 teaspoon ground cumin
- 1 cup brown uncooked rice
- 1 can (15 ounces) black beans, drained and rinsed
- 2 cups water
- Mushrooms and/or bell peppers, optional
- Cayenne pepper, if desired

Instructions

1. Heat oil over medium-high heat and sauté sausage and onion until onion becomes translucent.
2. Add the remaining ingredients and bring to boil over high heat. Reduce heat to low, cover and simmer for 40 minutes.

Tangy Yogurt Broiled Halibut

SERVINGS: 2
PREP TIME: 10 min.
TOTAL TIME: 20 min.

Ingredients

- 2 halibut fillets (5 ounces each)
- 1 cup non-fat plain yogurt
- 1 large clove garlic, peeled and crushed
- 1/4 teaspoon ground black pepper
- 1/4 cup freshly squeezed lemon juice
- 1/4 teaspoon salt

Instructions

1. Preheat broiler.
2. In a small bowl, combine yogurt, lemon juice, garlic, salt and pepper. Mix well.
3. Line a broiler pan with foil and place fish on top with the skin side down. Spread half of yogurt sauce over fish. Place fish 4 inches under broiler and cook for 10 minutes, or until fish flakes easily with a fork and topping is golden.
4. Serve warm with the rest of the yogurt sauce on the side.

Mediterranean-Style Grilled Salmon

SERVINGS: 4
PREP TIME: 10 min.
TOTAL TIME: 25 min.

Ingredients

- 4 tablespoons chopped fresh basil
- 1 tablespoon chopped fresh parsley
- 1 tablespoon minced garlic
- 2 tablespoons lemon juice
- 4 salmon fillets (5 ounces each)
- Black pepper, to taste
- 4 green olives, chopped
- 4 thin slices lemon

Instructions

1. Lightly coat grill rack or broiler pan with cooking spray and place cooking rack 4 to 6 inches from the heat source.
2. Preheat a gas grill or broiler.
3. Combine basil, parsley, minced garlic and lemon juice in a small bowl.
4. Spray fillets with cooking spray and sprinkle with black pepper. Top each with equal amounts of the basil-garlic mixture.
5. Place fillets herb-side down on grill over high heat. When edges turn white, turn fillets over and place on aluminium foil, about 3 to 4 minutes. Move to a cooler part of grill or reduce the heat. Grill until the opaque throughout when tested with the tip of a knife, about 4 more minutes.
6. Remove salmon and place on warmed plates. Garnish with green olives and lemon slices.

Chicken with Oranges and Avocados

SERVINGS: 4
PREP/TOTAL TIME: 35 min. + refrigeration

Ingredients

- 1 cup low-fat yogurt
- 1/4 cup minced red onion
- 1 tablespoon honey
- salt and ground black pepper, to taste
- 4 boneless skinless chicken breasts (4-6 ounce each)

Garnish

- 1 avocado
- 1/4 cup fresh lime juice
- 2 oranges, peeled and sectioned
- 2 tablespoon chopped cilantro
- 1 small red onion, thinly sliced

Instructions

1. In a large bowl, combine all the ingredients except the chicken and garnish. Add chicken to the mix and coat evenly. Cover and refrigerate for half an hour.
2. Preheat the grill or broiler.
3. Remove the chicken from the marinade. Sprinkle with salt and pepper.
4. Place chicken on the grill or under the broiler. Cook until juices run clear.
5. While the chicken is cooking, peel, core and chop the avocado and combine it with the lime juice quickly. Add oranges, onion and cilantro.
6. Season with salt and serve on top of chicken.

Lime and Cilantro Tilapia Tacos

SERVINGS: 2
PREP TIME: 10 min.
TOTAL TIME: 35 min.

Ingredients

- 1 pound tilapia filets, rinsed and patted dry
- 1 teaspoon olive oil
- 1 small onion, chopped
- 4 cloves garlic, finely minced
- 2 jalapeno peppers, chopped, and seeds removed
- 2 cups diced tomatoes
- 1/4 cup fresh cilantro, chopped
- 3 tablespoons lime juice
- Salt and pepper, to taste
- 8 5-inch white corn tortillas
- 1 medium avocado, sliced into 8 slices
- 1 cup shredded cabbage
- Lime wedges and fresh chopped cilantro, for garnish
- 4 tablespoons low-fat or fat free sour cream, optional

Instructions

1. Heat olive oil in a skillet. Sauté onion until translucent. Add garlic and mix well.
2. Place tilapia in skillet and cook until the flesh begins to flake.
3. Add jalapeno peppers, tomatoes, cilantro and lime juice.
4. Sauté over medium-high heat for about 5 minutes, breaking up the fish and mixing well.
5. Season to taste with salt and pepper.
6. Heat tortillas on a skillet on each side to warm for a few minutes.
7. Serve 1/4 cup of fish on each warmed tortilla with two avocado slices.
8. Split 1/4 cup of shredded cabbage and 1 tablespoon of low-fat or fat free sour cream between 2 tacos, if using.
9. Garnish with fresh chopped cilantro and lime wedges.

Sesame Baked Chicken Tenders

SERVINGS: 4
PREP TIME: 10 min.
TOTAL TIME: 25 min.

Ingredients

- 16 ounces chicken tenderloins
- 2 teaspoons sesame oil
- 2 teaspoons low sodium soy sauce
- 6 tablespoons toasted sesame seeds
- 1/2 teaspoon coarse salt
- 4 tablespoons breadcrumbs (no salt added)
- olive oil spray

Instructions

1. Preheat oven to 425°F (220°C). Spray a baking sheet with non-stick oil spray or parchment paper.
2. In a bowl, combine sesame oil and soy sauce.
3. In a separate bowl, combine sesame seeds, salt, and panko.
4. Place chicken in with the oil and soy sauce, and then place into sesame seed mix to coat well.
5. Place on baking sheet and lightly spray top of the chicken with oil spray. Bake 8-10 minutes. Turn and cook another 5 minutes or until cooked through.

Spicy Pork with Sweet Potatoes and Apples

SERVINGS: 4
PREP TIME: 15 min.
TOTAL TIME: 55 min.

Ingredients

- 3/4 cup apple cider
- 1/4 cup apple cider vinegar
- 2 tablespoons maple syrup
- 1/4 teaspoon smoked paprika
- 1 teaspoon grated fresh ginger or 1/4 teaspoon dried ginger
- 1 teaspoon ground black pepper
- 2 teaspoons vegetable oil
- 1 (12 ounce) pork tenderloin
- 1 large sweet potato, cut into 1/4 to 1/2-inch cubes
- 1 large apple, cut into 1/2 inch cubes

Instructions

1. Preheat oven to 375°F (190°C).
2. In a medium bowl, combine apple cider, apple cider vinegar, maple syrup, smoked paprika, ginger, and black pepper. Set aside.
3. Heat oil over medium-high heat in a large ovenproof sauté pan with a lid. Once oil starts to smoke, reduce heat to medium and gently place pork in pan. Cook, and turn until all sides are well browned, about 8 to 12 minutes. Remove pan from heat.
4. Place sweet potatoes around pork and pour apple cider mix over the tenderloin. Cover and bake for 20 minutes. Roast until instant-read thermometer inserted into the thickest part of the tenderloin reads 145–150°F (65°C).
5. Turn sweet potatoes and place apple quarters around pork. Bake uncovered for another 5 to 10 minutes, or until tenderloin registers 170°F (75°C). Remove pork, apples, and sweet potatoes from roasting pan. Let pork stand for 10 minutes before slicing.

6. As pork is resting, reduce cider mix to about a 1/4 cup. Slice roasted pork into 1/2 thick pieces. Serve with the sweet potatoes and apples and pour reduced cider over everything on the plate.

Glazed Turkey Breast with Fruit Stuffing

SERVINGS: 12
PREP TIME: 15 min.
TOTAL TIME: 2 1/2 hours

Ingredients

- 1-5 pound whole, bone-in turkey breast, thawed

Rub:

- 2 tablespoons fresh rosemary, chopped
- 2 tablespoons fresh thyme leaves, chopped
- 2 tablespoons olive oil

Stuffing:

- 1 small onion, thinly sliced
- 1 apple, peeled and thinly sliced
- 1 pear, peeled and thinly sliced
- 1/4 cup dried cranberries (or raisins)

Glaze:

- 2 cups (divided) apple juice
- 1 tablespoon brown sugar
- 1 tablespoon brown mustard
- 1 tablespoon olive oil

Instructions

1. Preheat oven to 325°F (165°C). Place turkey breast in a roasting pan, skin side up, on a rack.
2. In a small bowl, make a paste by combining the herbs and the olive oil. Loosen the skin from the meat with your fingers by making two deep pockets between skin and meat. Smear half the paste on the meat. Spread paste evenly over the top of the skin.

3. In another small bowl, mix the sliced onions and fruit. Stuff each pocket with the mixture.
4. Pour 1 cup of apple juice into the bottom of the roasting pan. Roast turkey breast for 1 hour 45 minutes to 2 hours, or until the skin is golden brown and a thermometer reads 165°F (73°C) when inserted into the thickest areas of the breast. If skin over-browns, cover breast loosely with aluminium foil.
5. In a sauce pan, combine remaining cup of apple juice, brown sugar, mustard and olive oil. Heat to boil. Reduce heat and simmer until it has thickened and reduced in volume to about 3/4 cup. Use to baste the turkey during the last half hour of cooking.
6. When turkey is done, cover with foil and allow to rest at room temperature for 15 minutes.
7. Carve, serve and spoon remaining glaze over the turkey.

Pork Chops with Black Currant Sauce

SERVINGS: 6
PREP TIME: 10 min.
TOTAL TIME: 30 min.

Ingredients

- 1/4 cup black currant jam
- 2 tablespoons Dijon mustard
- 2 teaspoons olive oil
- 6 center cut pork loin chops (4 ounces each), trimmed of all visible fat
- 1/3 cup wine vinegar
- 1/8 teaspoon freshly ground black pepper
- 6 orange slices

Instructions

1. In a small bowl, whisk together jam and mustard.
2. In a large non-stick frying pan, heat olive oil over medium-high heat. Add pork chops and cook, until browned on both sides, about 5 minutes on each side. Top each pork chop with 1 tablespoon of the jam-mustard mix. Cover and cook for 2 more minutes. Transfer to warmed plates.
3. Cool frying pan to a warm, but not hot, temperature. Pour wine vinegar into pan and stir to remove the bits of pork and jam. Pour vinegar sauce over each pork chop. Sprinkle with pepper and garnish with orange slices.
4. Serve immediately.

Honey Mustard Grilled Chicken with Toasted Almonds

SERVINGS: 4
PREP TIME: 10 min.
TOTAL TIME: 30 min.

Ingredients

- 1/4 cup Dijon mustard
- 3 teaspoon honey
- 1 teaspoon lemon juice
- 1 clove garlic, crushed
- 4 boneless, skinless chicken breasts
- 1/4 cup sliced almonds, toasted

Instructions

1. Preheat grill or broiler.
2. In a small bowl, combine mustard, honey, lemon juice, and garlic.
3. Brush chicken with the honey mustard sauce on both sides.
4. Grill or broil 6 inches from heat source for 10-15 minutes, occasionally turning and brushing with additional sauce; except for last 5 minutes. Discard remaining honey mustard sauce.
5. Sprinkle with almonds and serve.

Grilled Pesto Shrimp Skewers

SERVINGS: 7
PREP TIME: 20 min.
TOTAL TIME: 30 min. + refrigeration

Ingredients

- 1 cup fresh basil leaves, chopped
- 1 clove garlic, peeled
- 1/4 cup grated Parmigiano Reggiano cheese
- 3 tablespoons olive oil
- 1 1/2 pounds (weight after peeling) jumbo shrimp, peeled and deveined
- Salt and pepper, to taste
- 7 wooden skewers

Instructions

1. Pulse basil, garlic, parmesan cheese, salt and pepper in a food processor until smooth. Slowly add oil during pulsing. In a bowl, combine raw shrimp with pesto. Cover and marinate in the refrigerator for a few hours.
2. Soak wooden skewers in water for at least 20 minutes (or just use metal ones). Place the shrimp on skewers
3. Heat a grill pan over medium-low heat. Spray lightly with olive oil. Place shrimp on the grill and cook until they are pink on the bottom, about 3-4 minutes. Turn and cook until shrimp is opaque and cooked, about 3-4 more minutes.

Grilled Pork Fajitas

SERVINGS: 8
PREP TIME: 10 min.
TOTAL TIME: 25 min.

Ingredients

- 1 tablespoon chili powder
- 1/2 teaspoon oregano
- 1/2 teaspoon paprika
- 1/4 teaspoon ground coriander
- 1/4 teaspoon garlic powder
- 1 pound pork tenderloin, cut into strips 1/2 inch wide and 2 inches long
- 1 small onion, sliced
- 8 whole-wheat flour tortillas, about 8 inches in diameter, warmed in microwave
- 1/2 cup shredded sharp cheddar cheese
- 4 medium tomatoes, diced
- 4 cups shredded lettuce
- 1 cup salsa

Instructions

1. Heat a gas grill or broiler to medium-high heat or 400°F (200°C).
2. In a small bowl, combine and stir the chili powder, oregano, paprika, coriander and garlic powder. Coat the pork pieces completely in the seasonings.
3. In a cast-iron pan or grill basket, place the pork strips and onions. Grill or broil at medium-high heat until browned on all sides, about 5 minutes, turning several times.
4. Spread an equal amount of pork strips and onions on each tortilla. Top each with 1 tablespoon cheese, 2 tablespoons tomatoes, 1/2 cup shredded lettuce and 2 tablespoons salsa.
5. Fold in both sides of each tortilla, and roll to close.
6. Serve immediately.

Southeast Asian Baked Salmon

SERVINGS: 2
PREP TIME: 10 min.
TOTAL TIME: 35 min. + marinating

Ingredients

- 1/2 cup pineapple juice, no sugar added
- 2 garlic cloves, minced
- 1 teaspoon low-sodium soy sauce
- 1/4 teaspoon ground ginger
- 2 salmon fillets, 4 ounces each
- 1/4 teaspoon sesame oil
- Freshly ground black pepper, to taste
- 1 cup diced fresh fruit, such as pineapple, mango and papaya

Instructions

1. Add pineapple juice, garlic, soy sauce and ginger in a small bowl. Stir and evenly combine. In a small baking dish, arrange salmon fillets. Pour pineapple juice mix on top. Place in refrigerator and marinate for an hour. Turn the salmon occasionally as needed.
2. Heat oven to 375°F (190°C).
3. Lightly coat two squares of aluminium foil with cooking spray. Place marinated salmon fillets on aluminium foil. Drizzle each fillet with 1/8 teaspoon sesame oil. Sprinkle with pepper and top with 1/2 cup diced fruit on each. Wrap foil around the salmon and fold to seal edges. Bake about 10 minutes on each side, until fish is opaque throughout when cut with a knife.
4. Transfer salmon to individual plates and immediately serve.

Grilled Snapper Curry

SERVINGS: 4
PREP TIME: 10 min.
TOTAL TIME: 25 min.

Ingredients

- 1/2 teaspoon coconut extract
- 1 teaspoon black pepper
- 1/2 teaspoon fennel seed
- 1 tablespoon turmeric
- 1 teaspoon coriander
- 1 teaspoon cumin
- 1 teaspoon paprika
- 1 cup soy or skim milk
- 1 teaspoon corn-starch
- 1 teaspoon canola oil
- 2 tablespoons fresh ginger, minced
- 1 poblano pepper, sliced
- 2 cups sliced bok choy
- 2 cups sliced celery
- 1 cup sliced red bell pepper
- 1 cup sliced onion
- 2 cloves garlic, minced
- 4 six-ounce red snapper fillets

Instructions

1. Mix coconut extract and spices with milk and corn-starch. Set aside.
2. Place large skillet on medium-high heat. Add oil and sauté vegetables for a few minutes, until browned and vegetables are soft. Add milk and spice mixture to pan and stir. Heat gently, but do not boil. Remove from heat.
3. Broil or grill snapper until cooked or it reaches a temperature of 145°F (65°C).
4. Serve each fillet with 1 1/2 cups of vegetables and sauce.

Roasted Salmon with Maple Glaze

SERVINGS: 6
PREP TIME: 10 min.
TOTAL TIME: 45 min.

Ingredients

- 1/4 cup maple syrup
- 1 garlic clove, minced
- 1/4 cup balsamic vinegar
- 2 pounds salmon, cut into 6 equal-sized fillets
- 1/4 teaspoon kosher or sea salt
- 1/8 teaspoon fresh cracked black pepper
- Fresh mint or parsley for garnish

Instructions

1. Preheat oven to 450°F (230°C). Lightly coat a baking pan with cooking spray.
2. Mix together the maple syrup, garlic and balsamic vinegar in a small saucepan over low heat. Heat until hot and then remove from heat. Pour half of mix into a small bowl for basting, and reserve the rest for later.
3. Pat salmon dry. Place skin-side down on baking sheet. Brush salmon with the maple syrup mix. Bake about 10 minutes, and brush again with maple syrup mix, and bake for 5 more minutes. Continue to baste and bake until fish flakes easily, about 20 to 25 minutes in total.
4. Transfer salmon to plates.
5. Sprinkle with salt and black pepper, and top with reserved maple syrup mix. Garnish with fresh mint or parsley and serve immediately.

Spinach, Shrimp and Feta with Tuscan White Beans

SERVINGS: 4
PREP TIME: 5 min.
TOTAL TIME: 15 min.

Ingredients

- 2 tablespoons olive oil
- 1 pound large shrimp, peeled and deveined
- 1 medium onion, chopped
- 4 cloves garlic, minced
- 2 teaspoons chopped fresh sage
- 2 tablespoons balsamic vinegar
- 1/2 cup low sodium, fat-free chicken broth
- 15 ounce can no-salt added cannellini beans, rinsed and drained
- 5 cups baby spinach
- 1 1/2 ounce crumbled reduced-fat feta cheese

Instructions

1. In a large non-stick skillet, heat 1 teaspoon oil over medium-high heat. Cook shrimp until opaque, about 2 to 3 minutes. Transfer to a plate.
2. Heat remaining oil over medium-high heat and add onion, garlic and sage. Cook for 4 minutes occasionally stirring until golden. Stir in vinegar and cook 30 seconds.
3. Add broth, bring to a boil and cook 2 minutes. Stir in beans and spinach and cook about 2 to 3 minutes, until the spinach wilts. Remove from heat and stir in shrimp.
4. Top with feta cheese and divide in 4 bowls.

_D_ESSERTS

Red, White, and Blue Fruit Skewers and Cheesecake Dip

SERVINGS: 24
PREP/TOTAL TIME: 20 min.

Ingredients

Cheesecake dipping sauce:

- 4 ounces 1/3 less fat cream cheese, softened
- 1 cup fat free Greek yogurt
- 1 teaspoon vanilla extract
- 1/4 cup sugar

Skewers:

- 14 ounces angel food cake, cut into 1-inch cubes
- 72-84 medium strawberries (about 3 1/2 pounds), stems removed
- 1 pint blueberries
- 24-28 skewers

Instructions

1. Combine cream cheese with yogurt, vanilla and sugar in a medium bowl. Mix until sugar dissolves and set aside.
2. Thread 3 strawberries and 2 cubes of cake onto each skewer. Alternate between strawberries and cake. Finish each skewer with 3 blueberries and place finished skewers on a platter.
3. Refrigerate skewers and dip until ready to serve.

Honey and Yogurt Grilled Peaches

SERVINGS: 4
PREP TIME: 5 min.
TOTAL TIME: 10 min.

Ingredients

- 2 large ripe peaches, cut in half (pit removed)
- 1/4 cup fat free vanilla Greek yogurt
- 1/8 teaspoon cinnamon
- 2 tablespoons honey

Instructions

1. Heat grill to low heat.
2. Grill peaches, covered on low or indirect heat about 2-4 minutes on each side or until soft.
3. In a small bowl combine yogurt and cinnamon.
4. When the peaches are cooked, drizzle with honey and top each with 1 tablespoon of yogurt.

Blackberry Cinnamon Ginger Iced Tea

SERVINGS: 7
PREP TIME: 5 min.
TOTAL TIME: 20 min.

Ingredients

- 6 cups water
- 12 blackberry herbal tea bags
- 8 cinnamon sticks (3-inch-long)
- 1 tablespoon minced fresh ginger
- 1 cup unsweetened cranberry juice
- Sugar, to taste
- Ice cubes, crushed

Instructions

1. Heat water in a large saucepan, but avoid boiling. Add tea bags, two cinnamon sticks and ginger. Remove from heat, cover and steep for about 15 minutes.
2. Pass mix through a sieve into a pitcher. Add juice and sweetener to taste. Refrigerate until cold.
3. To serve, fill six tall glasses with crushed ice. Pour tea over the top of ice and garnish with cinnamon sticks.
4. Serve immediately.

Apples and Cream Shake

SERVINGS: 4
PREP/TOTAL TIME: 5 min.

Ingredients

- 2 cups vanilla low-fat ice cream
- 1 cup unsweetened applesauce
- 1/4 teaspoon ground cinnamon or apple pie spice
- 1 cup fat-free skim milk

Instructions.

1. In a blender, combine low-fat ice cream, applesauce and cinnamon or apple pie spice. Cover and blend until smooth.
2. Add fat-free skim milk. Cover and blend until well-mixed.
3. Pour into glasses. Sprinkle each serving with an additional cinnamon, if desired.
4. Serve immediately.

Fruited Rice Pudding

SERVINGS: 8
PREP TIME: 10 min.
TOTAL TIME: 1 hour 15 min.

Ingredients

- 2 cups water
- 1 cup long-grain rice
- 4 cups evaporated fat-free milk
- 1/2 cup brown sugar
- 1/2 teaspoon lemon zest
- 1 teaspoon vanilla extract
- 6 egg whites
- 1/4 cup crushed pineapple
- 1/4 cup raisins
- 1/4 cup chopped apricots

Instructions

1. Bring 2 cups of water to a boil in a medium saucepan. Add rice and cook for about 10 minutes. Pour into a colander and thoroughly drain.
2. In the same saucepan, add the evaporated milk and brown sugar, cooking until hot. Add the cooked rice, lemon zest and vanilla extract. Simmer over low heat until the mix is thick and rice is tender, about 30 minutes Remove from the heat and cool down.
3. In a small bowl whisk the egg whites together. Pour into the rice mix. Add pineapple, raisins and apricots. Stir until blended.
4. Preheat oven to 325°F (165°C). Lightly coat a baking dish with cooking spray.
5. Spoon pudding and fruit mix into the baking dish. Bake until the pudding is set, about 20 minutes.
6. Serve warm or cold.

SNACKS AND SIDES

Sweet and Spicy Roasted Red Pepper Hummus

SERVINGS: 8
PREP/TOTAL TIME: 10 min.

Ingredients

- 1 (15 ounce) can garbanzo (chickpeas) beans, drained
- 1 (4 ounce) jar roasted red peppers
- 3 tablespoons lemon juice
- 1 1/2 tablespoons tahini
- 1 clove garlic, minced
- 1/2 teaspoon ground cumin
- 1/2 teaspoon cayenne pepper
- 1/4 teaspoon salt
- 1 tablespoon chopped fresh parsley

Instructions

1. Puree chickpeas, red peppers, lemon juice, tahini, garlic, cumin, cayenne, and salt in an electric blender or food processor. Process using long pulses until smooth and slightly fluffy. Scrape the mixture off the sides between pulses. Transfer to a serving bowl and refrigerate at least an hour.
2. Return to room temperature before serving. Sprinkle with the chopped parsley before serving.

Chipotle Spiced Shrimp

SERVINGS: 4
PREP TIME:
TOTAL TIME:

Ingredients

- 3/4 pound uncooked shrimp, peeled and deveined (about 48 shrimps)
- 2 tablespoons tomato paste
- 1 1/2 teaspoons water
- 1/2 teaspoon extra-virgin olive oil
- 1/2 teaspoon minced garlic
- 1/2 teaspoon chipotle chili powder
- 1/2 teaspoon fresh oregano, chopped

Instructions

1. Rinse shrimp in cold water and pat dry with a paper towel. Set aside.
2. In a small bowl whisk together tomato paste, water and oil. Mix in garlic, chili powder and oregano.
3. Using a brush, spread the marinade mix on both sides of the shrimp. Place in the refrigerator.
4. Preheat a gas grill or broiler. Lightly coat grill rack or broiler pan with cooking spray. Position the cooking rack 4 to 6 inches from the heat source.
5. Put shrimp in grill basket or on skewers and place on the grill. Turn shrimp after 3 to 4 minutes.

Lemon Glaze

SERVINGS: 4
PREP/ TOTAL TIME: 5 min.

Ingredients

- 1 teaspoon lemon or lime juice
- 1 teaspoon grated lemon or lime zest
- 1/2 cup unsalted chicken broth
- 1 tablespoon chopped parsley
- 1 tablespoon sugar
- 2 teaspoons corn-starch

Instructions

1. Combine all the ingredients in a microwavable bowl. Whisk and mix evenly. Microwave on high until clear and thickened, about 1 to 2 minutes.
2. Serve immediately with chicken, fish, or vegetables.

Maple Mustard Kale with Turkey Bacon

SERVINGS: 4
PREP TIME: 5 min.
TOTAL TIME: 10 min.

Ingredients

- 1 tsp olive oil
- 1/2 large onion, sliced
- 3 strips turkey bacon cut crosswise into strips
- 1 bunch kale
- 1 tablespoon whole grained mustard
- 1 teaspoon apple cider vinegar
- 1 tablespoon 100% pure maple syrup

Instructions

1. Remove tough ribs from kale. Cut into bite-size pieces. Wash well and pat dry.
2. Heat a large sauté pan over medium heat. Add olive oil, onions and turkey bacon and sauté about 8 minutes or until browned.
3. Add washed kale and cook until wilted, stirring occasionally, for about 4 minutes.
4. Combine whole grain mustard, apple cider vinegar and pure maple syrup, in a small bowl.
5. When kale is wilted and tender, drizzle mustard mix over the kale and stir to combine. Heat for about 1 minute. Serve warm.

Garlic and Kale with Black-Eyed Peas

SERVINGS: 6
PREP TIME: 10 min.
TOTAL TIME: 30 min.

Ingredients

- 1 1/2 pounds kale, washed and drained
- 1 teaspoon olive or other vegetable oil
- 1 teaspoon chopped fresh garlic, or more to taste
- Pinch of dried red pepper flakes
- 2 cup canned black-eyed peas, drained (or cooked from dry)
- 1 teaspoon cider vinegar, to taste

Instructions

1. Pull kale leaves from tough stems. Discard stems and chop leaves into one-inch pieces.
2. Place two inches of water in a large pot and boil. Add kale, cover and cook 15 to 20 minutes or until tender, stirring occasionally. Drain, reserving water for soup if desired.
3. Heat a large non-stick skillet over medium-low heat. Add oil and garlic. Cook garlic while stirring, about 2 minutes or until it begins to sizzle.
4. Add black-eyed peas and red pepper flakes and cook about 3 minutes or until heated through, stirring occasionally.
5. Add kale and stir to combine over low heat.
6. Add cider vinegar just before serving.

Sweet and Spicy Snack Mix

SERVINGS: 4
PREP TIME: 5 min.
TOTAL TIME: 50 min.

Ingredients

- butter-flavored cooking spray
- 2 cans (15 ounces each) garbanzos beans (chickpeas), rinsed, drained and patted dry
- 2 cups wheat squares cereal
- 1 cup dried pineapple chunks
- 1 cup raisins
- 2 tablespoons honey
- 2 tablespoons Worcestershire sauce
- 1 teaspoon garlic powder
- 1/2 teaspoon chili powder

Instructions

1. Preheat oven to 350°F (175°C). Lightly coat a 15 1/2-inch-by-10 1/2-inch baking sheet with butter-flavored cooking spray or grease.
2. Spray a heavy skillet generously with butter-flavored cooking spray. Add garbanzos and cook over medium heat. Stir frequently for about 10 minutes or until beans begin to brown. Transfer to the prepared baking sheet. Spray beans lightly with cooking spray. Bake about 20 minutes, stirring frequently until beans are crisp.
3. Lightly coat a roasting pan with butter-flavored cooking spray. Add cereal, pineapple, raisins and roasted garbanzos to pan. Stir to evenly mix.
4. In a large measuring cup combine honey, Worcestershire sauce and spices. Stir to evenly mix. Pour over the snack mix and gently toss. Spray mix again with cooking spray. Bake for 10 to 15 minutes, stirring occasionally to keep from burning.
5. Remove from oven and let cool.

Baked Pears with Walnuts and Honey

SERVINGS: 4
PREP TIME: 15 min.
TOTAL TIME: 45 min.

Ingredients

- 2 large ripe pears
- 1/4 teaspoon ground cinnamon
- 2 teaspoon honey
- 1/4 cup crushed walnuts

Instructions

1. Preheat the oven to 350°F (175°C).
2. Cut pears in half and place on a baking sheet and scoop out the seeds.
3. Sprinkle with cinnamon. Top with walnuts and drizzle 1/2 teaspoon honey over each one.
4. Bake in the oven 30 minutes.
5. Let cool and serve.

Classic Boston Baked Beans

SERVINGS: 12
PREP TIME: 15 min.
TOTAL TIME: 6 hours

Ingredients

- 2 cups dried small, white beans (navy beans), rinsed, soaked overnight and drained
- 4 cups water
- 2 bay leaves
- 3/4 teaspoon salt, divided
- 1 yellow onion, chopped
- 1/2 cup light molasses
- 1 1/2 tablespoons dry mustard
- 3 strips thick-cut bacon, cut into 1/2-inch pieces

Instructions

1. In a Dutch oven or a large ovenproof pot with a tight-fitting lid, combine beans, water, bay leaves and 1/2 teaspoon of the salt over high heat. Bring to a boil. Reduce heat to low, partially cover and simmer for 65 to 75 minutes until beans have softened but are firm. Remove from heat and discard bay leaves. Don't drain beans.
2. Preheat oven to 350°F (175°C).
3. Stir the onion, molasses, mustard, bacon and the remaining 1/4 teaspoon salt into the beans. Cover and bake for 4 1/2 to 5 hours until beans are tender and coated with a light syrup. Check periodically to make sure the beans don't dry out, stirring and adding hot water when needed.

Grilled Mango Chutney

SERVINGS: 6
PREP TIME: 10 min.
TOTAL TIME: 20 min.

Ingredients

- 1 mango, peeled and pitted
- 1/4 cup sugar
- 1/4 cup chopped red onion
- 2 tablespoons cider vinegar
- 2 tablespoons finely chopped green bell pepper
- 1 tablespoon grated fresh ginger
- 1/2 teaspoon ground ginger
- 1/8 teaspoon ground cloves
- 1/4 teaspoon chopped fresh rosemary

Instructions

1. Preheat a gas grill or broiler. Position the cooking rack 4 to 6 inches from heat source.
2. Arrange mango on the grill rack or broiler pan. Broil on medium heat, about 2 to 3 minutes on each side, turning often, until softened and slightly browned.
3. Remove mango from the grill and let cool for a few minutes.
4. Chop small chunks and serve.

Sherried Mushroom Sauce

SERVINGS: 12
PREP TIME: 5 min.
TOTAL TIME: 20 min.

Ingredients

- 2 cups fat-free milk
- 2 teaspoons canola oil
- 1 small onion, diced
- 1 1/2 cups sliced fresh mushrooms
- 2 tablespoons all-purpose (plain) flour
- 1 tablespoon chopped chives
- Ground black pepper, to taste
- 1 teaspoon sherry (optional)

Instructions

1. Over low heat, warm milk in a small saucepan.
2. Heat canola oil in a non-stick skillet over medium heat. Add onions and sauté for 3 minutes. Add sliced mushrooms and sauté another 3 minutes. Stir in flour and cook another 2 to 3 minutes. Whisk in warmed milk and stirring frequently until thickened, about 3 minutes. Add chives, pepper and sherry, if desired.
3. Keep mushroom sauce warmed over low heat until served.

Bulgur Stuffing with Dried Cranberries and Hazelnuts

SERVINGS: 10
PREP TIME: 15 min.
TOTAL TIME: 45 min.

Ingredients

- 1 tablespoons olive oil
- 3 cups chopped onions (2 large)
- 1 cup chopped celery (2-3 stalks)
- 1 clove garlic, minced
- 1/2 teaspoon ground cinnamon
- 1/4 teaspoon ground allspice
- 2 cups bulgur, rinsed
- 3 cups reduced-sodium chicken broth
- 1 bay leaf
- 1/4 teaspoon salt
- 2/3 cup dried cranberries
- 1/4 cup orange juice
- 2/3 cup chopped hazelnuts (about 2 ounces) roasted
- 1/2 cup chopped fresh flat leaf parsley
- 1/4 teaspoon fresh ground black pepper

Instructions

1. Heat oil over medium heat. Add onions and celery, cook for 5-8 minutes stirring often until softened.
2. Add garlic, cinnamon and allspice, cook for one minute while stirring.
3. Add bulgur and stir for a few seconds, add broth, bay leaf and salt, bring to a simmer.
4. Reduce heat to low, cover and simmer 15-20 minutes until bulgur is tender and liquid is absorbed.
5. Meanwhile, combine dried cranberries and orange juice in a small microwave safe container. Cover with plastic wrap and microwave on high for 2 minutes. Let cranberries rest while covered, for another minute or two.

6. When bulgur has cooked, discard bay leaf, add cranberries with orange juice, toasted hazelnuts, parsley and pepper. Fluff with a fork and serve.

Southwest Potato Skins

SERVINGS: 6
PREP TIME: 10 min.
TOTAL TIME: 30 min.

Ingredients

- 6 large baking potatoes
- 1 teaspoon olive oil
- 1 teaspoon chili powder
- 1/8 teaspoon Tabasco sauce
- 6 slices turkey bacon, cooked until crisp, chopped
- 1 medium tomato, diced
- 2 tablespoons sliced green onions
- 1/2 cup shredded cheddar cheese

Instructions

1. Preheat the oven to 450°F (230°F). Lightly coat a baking sheet with cooking spray.
2. Scrub potatoes and prick each several times with a fork. Microwave uncovered on high about 10 minutes or until tender. Remove potatoes from microwave and place on a wire rack to cool. When cool, cut each in half lengthwise. Scoop out the flesh, leaving about 1/4 inch of the flesh attached to the skin. (Save potato flesh for something else.)
3. Whisk together olive oil, chili powder and hot sauce in a small bowl. Brush olive oil mix on the insides of the potato skins. Cut each half of the potato skin in half crosswise again. Place potatoes on baking sheet.
4. Mix the turkey bacon, tomato and onions in a small bowl. Fill each potato skin with this mix and sprinkle with cheese.
5. Bake about 10 minutes or until cheese is melted and the potato skins are heated through.
6. Serve immediately.

Shrimp ceviche

SERVINGS: 8
PREP/TOTAL TIME: 10 min. + refrigeration

Ingredients

- 1/2 pound raw shrimp, cut in 1/4-inch pieces
- 2 lemons, zest and juice
- 2 limes, zest and juice
- 2 tablespoons olive oil
- 2 teaspoons cumin
- 1/2 cup diced red onion
- 1 cup diced tomato
- 2 tablespoons minced garlic
- 1 cup black beans, cooked
- 1/4 cup serrano chili pepper, diced and seeds removed
- 1 cup diced cucumber, peeled and seeded
- 1/4 cup chopped cilantro

Instructions

1. Place shrimp in a shallow pan and cover with juice from the lemon and lime. Reserving the zest. Refrigerate for at least 3 hours or until shrimp is firm and white.
2. In a separate bowl, mix remaining ingredients and set aside while shrimp is cooking in the fridge. When ready to serve, mix shrimp and citrus juice with remaining ingredients.
3. Serve with tortilla chips.

THANK YOU

Thank you for checking out the DASH Diet Cookbook. I hope you enjoyed these recipes as much as I have. I am always looking for feedback on how to improve, so if you have any questions, suggestions, or comments please send me an email at susan.evans.author@gmail.com. Also, if you enjoyed the book would you consider leaving on honest review? As a new author, they help me out in a big way. Thanks again, and have fun cooking!

Check out more cookbooks

Vegetarian Mediterranean Cookbook:
Over 50 recipes for appetizers, salads, dips, and main dishes

Quick & Easy Asian Vegetarian Cookbook:
Over 50 recipes for stir fries, rice, noodles, and appetizers

Vegetarian Slow Cooker Cookbook:
Over 75 recipes for meals, soups, stews, desserts, and sides

Quick & Easy Vegan Desserts Cookbook:
Over 80 delicious recipes for cakes, cupcakes, brownies, cookies, fudge, pies, candy, and so much more!

Quick & Easy Microwave Meals:
Over 50 recipes for breakfast, snacks, meals and desserts

Halloween Cookbook:
80 Ghoulish recipes for appetizers, meals, drinks, and desserts

Printed in Great Britain
by Amazon